# Pocket Guide to Radiation Oncology

# Pocket Guide to Radiation Oncology

**EDITORS**

**DANIEL D. CHAMBERLAIN, MD**
Adjunct Assistant Professor
University of Texas MD Anderson
Banner MD Anderson Cancer Center
Gilbert, Arizona

**JAMES B. YU, MD, MHS**
Associate Professor
Department of Therapeutic Radiology
Yale University School of Medicine
Cancer Outcomes, Public Policy, and Effectiveness Research
(COPPER) Center at Yale
New Haven, Connecticut

**ROY H. DECKER, MD, PhD**
Associate Professor
Residency Training Program Director
Department of Therapeutic Radiology
Yale University School of Medicine
New Haven, Connecticut

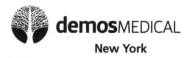
**demos**MEDICAL

**New York**

Visit our website at www.demosmedical.com

*ISBN:* 9781620700891
*e-book ISBN:* 9781617052651

*Acquisitions Editor:* David D'Addona
*Compositor:* diacriTech

Copyright © 2017 Springer Publishing Company.
Demos Medical Publishing is an imprint of Springer Publishing Company, LLC.

**Library of Congress Cataloging-in-Publication Data**

Names: Chamberlain, Daniel, editor. | Yu, James B., editor. | Decker, Roy H.,
    editor.
Title: Pocket guide to radiation oncology / [edited by] Daniel Chamberlain,
    James B. Yu, Roy H. Decker.
Description: New York : Demos Medical Publishing, [2016] | Includes
    bibliographical references and index.
Identifiers: LCCN 2016024472| ISBN 9781620700891 | ISBN 9781617052651 (ebook)
Subjects: | MESH: Neoplasms—radiotherapy | Radiation Oncology | Handbooks
Classification: LCC RC271.R3 | NLM QZ 39 | DDC 616.99/40642—dc23 LC record
available at https://lccn.loc.gov/2016024472

Special discounts on bulk quantities of Demos Medical Publishing books are available to corporations, professional associations, pharmaceutical companies, health
care organizations, and other qualifying groups. For details, please contact:

Special Sales Department
Demos Medical Publishing
11 West 42nd Street, 15th Floor, New York, NY 10036
Phone: 800-532-8663 or 212-683-0072; Fax: 212-941-7842
E-mail: specialsales@demosmedical.com

Printed in the United States of America by Gasch Printing.
16  17  18  19  20 / 5  4  3  2  1

"For our children"

# CONTENTS

# CONTRIBUTORS

**Sahaja Acharya, MD**
Department of Radiation Oncology
Washington University School of Medicine
St Louis, Missouri

**Aida Amado, ACNP-BC**
Banner MD Anderson Cancer Center
Gilbert, Arizona

**Sanjay Aneja, MD**
Department of Therapeutic Radiology
Yale School of Medicine
New Haven, Connecticut

**Andrew Bishop, MD**
Department of Radiation Oncology
The University of Texas MD Anderson Cancer Center
Houston, Texas

**Tomasz Bista, MS**
Banner MD Anderson Cancer Center
Gilbert, Arizona

**Trevor Bledsoe, MD**
Department of Therapeutic Radiology
Yale School of Medicine
New Haven, Connecticut

**Daniel D. Chamberlain, MD**
University of Texas MD Anderson
Banner MD Anderson Cancer Center
Gilbert, Arizona

**Linda Chen, MD**
Department of Radiation Oncology
The Johns Hopkins School of Medicine
Baltimore, Maryland

**Shari Damast, MD**
Department of Therapeutic Radiology
Yale School of Medicine
New Haven, Connecticut

**Roy H. Decker, MD, PhD**
Department of Therapeutic Radiology
Yale University School of Medicine
New Haven, Connecticut

**Adam Ferro, MD, MS**
Department of Radiation Oncology
The Johns Hopkins School of Medicine
Baltimore, Maryland

**B. Ashleigh Guadagnolo, MD**
Department of Radiation Oncology
The University of Texas MD Anderson Cancer Center
Houston, Texas

**Zach Guss, MD, MSc**
Department of Radiation Oncology
The Johns Hopkins School of Medicine
Baltimore, Maryland

**Skyler Johnson, MD**
Department of Therapeutic Radiology
Yale School of Medicine
New Haven, Connecticut

**Jacqueline Kelly, MD, MSc**
Department of Therapeutic Radiology
Yale School of Medicine
New Haven, Connecticut

**Ana Kiess, MD, PhD**
Department of Radiation Oncology
The Johns Hopkins School of Medicine
Baltimore, Maryland

**Adam Kole, MD, PhD**
Department of Therapeutic Radiology
Yale School of Medicine
New Haven, Connecticut

**Deborah A. Kuban, MD**
Department of Radiation Oncology
The University of Texas MD Anderson Cancer Center
Houston, Texas

**Rachit Kumar, MD**
Banner MD Anderson Cancer Center
Gilbert, Arizona

**Anna Likhacheva, MD**
Banner MD Anderson Cancer Center
Gilbert, Arizona;
Department of Radiation Oncology
The University of Texas MD Anderson Cancer Center
Houston, Texas

**Jerry T. Liu, MD**
Department of Radiation Oncology
Icahn School of Medicine at Mount Sinai
New York, New York

**Kimberly Lauren Johung, MD, PhD**
Department of Therapeutic Radiology
Yale School of Medicine
New Haven, Connecticut

**Brandon R. Mancini, MD**
Department of Therapeutic Radiology
Yale School of Medicine
New Haven, Connecticut

**Omar Mian, MD, PhD**
Department of Radiation Oncology
The Johns Hopkins School of Medicine
Baltimore, Maryland

**Meena Moran, MD**
Department of Therapeutic Radiology
Yale School of Medicine
New Haven, Connecticut

**Sabin B. Motwani, MD**
Rutgers Cancer Institute of New Jersey
New Brunswick, New Jersey

**Sameer Nath, MD**
Department of Therapeutic Radiology
Yale School of Medicine
New Haven, Connecticut

**Sarah Nicholas, MD**
Department of Radiation Oncology
The Johns Hopkins School of Medicine
Baltimore, Maryland

**Arti Parekh, MD**
Department of Radiation Oncology
The Johns Hopkins School of Medicine
Baltimore, Maryland

**Rahul R. Parikh, MD**
Department of Radiation Oncology
Robert Wood Johnson Medical School
New Brunswick, New Jersey

**Stephanie M. Perkins, MD**
Department of Radiation Oncology
Washington University School of Medicine
St Louis, Missouri

**James Y. Rao, MD**
Department of Radiation Oncology
Washington University School of Medicine
St Louis, Missouri

**Charles Rutter, MD**
Department of Therapeutic Radiology
Yale School of Medicine
New Haven, Connecticut

**Colette Shen, MD**
Department of Radiation Oncology
The Johns Hopkins School of Medicine
Baltimore, Maryland

**Neil Taunk, MD**
Department of Radiation Oncology
Memorial Sloan Kettering Cancer Center
New York, New York

**Ahmet Tunceroğlu, MD, PhD**
Department of Radiation Oncology
Robert Wood Johnson Medical School
New Brunswick, New Jersey

**Gary Walker, MD**
Banner MD Anderson Cancer Center
Gilbert, Arizona

**Debra Nana Yeboa, MD**
Department of Therapeutic Radiology
Yale School of Medicine
New Haven, Connecticut

**Melissa Young, MD, PhD**
Department of Therapeutic Radiology
Yale School of Medicine
New Haven, Connecticut

**James B. Yu, MD, MHS**
Department of Therapeutic Radiology
Yale University School of Medicine
Cancer Outcomes, Public Policy, and Effectiveness Research
(COPPER) Center at Yale
New Haven, Connecticut

# ABBREVIATIONS

| | |
|---|---|
| 3DCRT | 3D conformal radiation therapy |
| 4DCT | 4 Dimensional computed tomography |
| ABS | American Brachytherapy Society |
| ABVD | Adriamycin Bleomycin Vinblastine Dacarbazine |
| ADT | Androgen deprivation therapy |
| AFP | Alpha fetoprotein |
| ALCL | Anaplastic large cell lymphoma |
| AP | Anterior posterior |
| APR | Abdominoperitoneal resection |
| BCG | Bacillus Calmette-Guerin intravesicular therapy |
| BEACOPP | Bleomycin Etoposide Adriamycin Cyclophosphamide Oncovin (Vincristine) Procarbazine Prednisone |
| BID | Twice per day |
| BUN/Cr | Blood urea nitrogen/Creatinine |
| bPFS | Biochemical Progression Free Survival |
| C/A/P | Chest / Abdomen / Pelvis |
| CA125 | Cancer antigen 125 |
| CA19-9 | Carbohydrate antigen 19-9 (also called cancer antigen 19-9) |
| CBC | Complete blood count |
| CBCT | Cone beam computed tomography |
| CEA | Carcinoembryonic antigen |
| ChemoRT | Chemoradiation therapy |
| CLL/SLL | Chronic lymphocytic leukemia / small lymphocytic lymphoma |
| CMP | Comprehensive metabolic panel |
| CR | Complete response |
| CSF | Cerebrospinal fluid |
| CSI | Cranial spinal radiation therapy |
| CT | Computed tomography |
| CTV | Clinical target volume |
| CXR | Chest X-ray |
| D&C | Dilation and curettage |
| DFS | Disease free survival |
| DLBCL | Diffuse large B cell lymphoma |
| DM | Distant metastasis |
| DMFS | Distant metastasis free survival |

| DRE | Digital rectal exam |
|---|---|
| DSS | Disease specific survival |
| DVH | Dose volume histogram |
| D2cc | Dose for the most exposed 2cc of an organ |
| D90 | Minimum dose covering 90% of target |
| EBRT | External beam radiation therapy |
| EBV | Epstein-Barr Virus |
| ECE | Extracapsular extension |
| EFS | Event free survival |
| EGD | Esophagogastroduodenoscopy |
| EQD2 | Equivalent dose in 2 Gray per fraction |
| ERCP | Endoscopic retrograde cholangiopancreatography |
| ER/PR | Estrogen receptor / progesterone receptor |
| EUA | Exam under anesthesia |
| EUS | Endoscopic ultrasound |
| FFF | Freedom from failure |
| FFS | Failure free survival |
| FISH | Fluorescence in situ hybridization |
| FL | Follicular lymphoma |
| FNA | Fine needle aspiration |
| FOLFIRI | Folinic acid, Fluorouracil, Irinotecan |
| FOLFOX | Folinic acid, Fluorouracil, Oxaliplatin |
| fx | Fractions |
| GE | Gastroesophageal |
| GI | Gastrointestinal |
| GTR | Gross total resection |
| GTV | Gross tumor volume |
| Gy | Gray |
| H&P | History and physical |
| HCC | Hepatocellular carcinoma |
| HDR | High dose rate (brachytherapy) |
| HIV | Human immunodeficiency virus |
| HLA | Human leukocyte antigen |
| HPV | Human papilloma virus |
| HT | Hormonal therapy |
| IBTR | Ipsilateral breast tumor recurrence |
| ICRT | Intra-cavitary radiation therapy |
| IFRT | Involved field radiotherapy |
| IG-SRS | Image guided stereotactic radiosurgery |
| IGRT | Image guided radiation therapy |
| IHC | Immunohistochemistry |
| IMRT | Intensity modulated radiation therapy |
| IORT | Intraoperative radiotherapy |

| | |
|---|---|
| ITV | Internal tumor volume |
| IV | Intravenous |
| IVC | Inferior vena cava |
| IVRT | Intra-vaginal radiation therapy |
| KPS | Karnofsky Performance Status |
| LAR | Low anterior resection |
| LC | Local control |
| LDH | Lactate dehydrogenase |
| LDR | Low dose rate (brachytherapy) |
| LFTs | Liver function tests |
| LN | Lymph node |
| LP | Lumbar puncture |
| LRR | Local regional recurrence |
| LVSI | Lymphovascular invasion |
| MALT | Mucosa associated lymphoid tissue |
| MCL | Mantle cell lymphoma |
| MF | Mycosis fungoides |
| MRI | Magnetic resonance imaging |
| MZL | Marginal zone lymphoma |
| NED | No evidence of disease |
| NLPHL | Nodular lymphocyte-predominant Hodgkin lymphoma |
| NK | Natural killer |
| OAR | Organ at risk |
| OBS | Observation |
| OS | Overall survival |
| PA | Posterior anterior |
| PCFCL | Primary cutaneous follicular center lymphoma |
| PCMZL | Primary cutaneous marginal zone lymphoma |
| PCNSL | Primary CNS lymphoma |
| PCSS | Prostate cancer specific survival |
| PCTCL | Primary cutaneous T-Cell Lymphoma |
| PCV | Procarbazine CCNU and Vincristine |
| PET | Positron emission tomography |
| PFS | Progression free survival |
| PMBL/GZL | Primary mediastinal B-cell lymphoma / Gray zone lymphoma |
| PNET | Primitive neuroectodermal tumor |
| PO | By mouth |
| PSA | Prostate-specific antigen |
| PTCL | Peripheral T-cell lymphoma |
| PTV | Planning tumor volume |
| QD | Once per day |

| | |
|---|---|
| QoL | Quality of life |
| RANO | Response assessment in neuro-oncology |
| RCHOP | Rituximab cyclophosphamide doxorubicin vincristine prednisone |
| RFA | Radiofrequency ablation |
| RFS | Relapse free survival |
| RTOG | Radiation therapy oncology group |
| RP | Radical prostatectomy |
| RT | Radiation therapy |
| s/p | Status post |
| SBRT | Stereotactic body radiotherapy |
| SRS | Stereotactic radiosurgery |
| SRT | stereotactic radiotherapy |
| SS | Statistically Significant |
| SSD | Source to surface distance |
| SV | Seminal vesicles |
| TACE | Transcatheter arterial chemoembolization |
| TAH/BSO | Total abdominal hysterectomy / Bilateral Salpingo-oophorectomy |
| TH/BSO | Total hysterectomy / Bilateral Salpingo-oophorectomy |
| TID | Three times per day |
| TME | Total mesorectal excision |
| TSEBT | Total skin electron beam therapy |
| VEGF | Vascular endothelial growth factor |
| VMAT | Volumetric modulated arc therapy |
| VP | Ventriculoperitoneal |
| WART | Whole abdominal radiation therapy |
| WBRT | whole brain radiation therapy |
| WHO PS | World Health Organization Performance Status |
| WPRT | Whole pelvis radiation therapy |
| 32P | Phosphorus-32 |

# PREFACE

We first conceived of this project years ago when we were all residents putting together study sheets in preparation for eventual board certification exams. We imagined taking our painstakingly created study sheets and distributing them to our fellow residents and medical students, passing them out with a wink and a nod to colleagues around the country. As trainees, the idea of a "little black book" of radiation oncology that could be surreptitiously looked at before walking into a patient's room, or before being questioned by an attending physician in chart rounds, held great appeal.

Now that we are all older, grayer, and specialized, a rapid reference that allows for quick review of the existing standard of care and most relevant literature promises to save us time and energy, and reassurance that we won't put our feet in our mouths when covering tumor boards we don't normally cover, or staff satellites for our colleagues and see patients we don't usually see. In the era of quick curbside conversations and multitasking, this quick pocket-sized reference can be carried for a quick review between our children's activities instead of heavy textbooks often filled with esoteric topics and unnecessarily minutiae.

We hope that this text, *Pocket Guide to Radiation Oncology* will indeed reside in the pockets of our colleagues, trainees, and staff. We are indebted to the authors who have contributed their expertise to this text.

*Daniel D. Chamberlain, MD*
*James B. Yu, MD, MHS*
*Roy H. Decker, MD, PhD*

# 1: BRAIN METASTASIS

*Sabin B. Motwani, MD*

## WORKUP

### All Cases

- ▦ H&P (make note of age, performance status, neuro deficits, # of mets, presence of extracranial mets)
- ▦ MRI brain w/ and w/o contrast
- ▦ If solitary lesion, consider biopsy

### Considerations

- ▦ Disease-specific Graded Prognostic Assessment (DS-GPA) to assess prognosis (Sperduto et al., *JCO* 2012; DOI: 10.1200/JCO.2011.38.0527)
- ▦ Prognostic systems for radiosurgery: score index for radiosurgery (SIR), and basic score-brain metastasis (BS-BM) (Lorenzoni et al., *IJROBP* 2004; DOI: 10.1016/j.ijrobp.2004.02.017)

## TREATMENT RECOMMENDATIONS BY # OF METS, RESECTABILITY, AND PROGNOSIS

| | |
|---|---|
| Single metastasis, resectable, <4 cm, prognosis >3 months | Surgery → WBRT<br>OR WBRT → SRS<br>OR SRS alone<br>OR Surgery → SRS to resection cavity |
| Single metastasis, resectable, >4 cm, prognosis >3 months | Surgery → WBRT<br>OR Surgery → SRS to resection cavity ± WBRT |
| Single metastasis, unresectable, <4 cm, prognosis >3 months | SRS → WBRT<br>OR SRS alone |
| Single metastasis, unresectable, >4 cm, prognosis >3 months | WBRT<br>OR WBRT ± SRS if good response to WBRT<br>OR hypofractionated SRT |
| Multiple metastasis, all mets <4 cm, prognosis >3 months | WBRT → SRS<br>OR SRS alone<br>OR WBRT alone |

*(continued)*

(continued)

| Multiple metastasis, mets causing mass effect, prognosis >3 months | Surgery of met(s) causing mass effect → WBRT<br>OR surgery of met(s) causing mass effect → SRS ± WBRT |
| Poor prognosis <3 months, KPS <50, regardless # of mets | WBRT alone<br>OR palliative care alone<br>OR hospice |

Consider hippocampal sparing WBRT* or giving patients memantine while receiving WBRT.

## TECHNICAL CONSIDERATIONS

### Simulation

Simulate neutral head position and treat with aquaplast mask if whole brain. More robust immobilization and/or image guidance for enhanced precision if SRS treatment. Obtain thin-slice MRI (Stealth MRI) for SRS planning.

### Dose Prescription

- Whole brain: 30 Gy in 10 fx (most common in the United States)
    35 to 37.5 Gy in 14 to 15 fx
    20 Gy in 5 fx (most common worldwide)
- SRS: 20 to 24 Gy for mets ≤2 cm
    18 Gy for mets 2 cm < × ≤3 cm
    15 Gy for mets 3 cm < × ≤4 cm

For Gamma Knife, Rx prescription is typically to the 50% isodose line (IDL), and for Linac-SRS, Rx prescription is typically to the 80% IDL.

### Target Delineation

- Whole brain: typically flash 1.5 cm anteriorly, superiorly, and posteriorly. Inferior border: C1 or C2.
- Block is drawn to spare eye.

SRS: 1- to 2-mm margin around lesion or resection cavity.

### Treatment Planning

- Whole brain: opposed laterals*
- *For hippocampal-sparing WBRT, see Gondi et al., *IJROBP* 2010;78:1244–52 (DOI: 10.1016/j.ijrobp.2010.11.001).

## FOLLOW UP

MRI brain and H&P q2 to 3 months.

## SELECTED STUDIES

*Single Brain Met*

### Patchell II (Patchell, *JAMA* 1998; DOI: 10.1001/jama.280.17.1485)

95 patients. Complete resection verified by MRI. Randomized after surgery to WBRT or observation. WBRT dose 50.4 Gy over 5.5 weeks.

- Post-op WBRT reduced local recurrence (10% vs. 46%), distance recurrence (18% vs. 70%), and neurological death (14% vs. 44%).
- No change in overall survival (OS) or time patient remained functionally independent.

*Limited Brain Mets (1–3)*
*WBRT versus WBRT + SRS*

### RTOG 9508 (Andrews, *Lancet* 2004; DOI: 10.1016/S0140-6736(04)16250-8)

331 patients. Lesions <4 cm; RPA I (26%) and II (74%) randomized to WBRT (37.5 Gy in 15 fx) alone versus WBRT + SRS. SRS 18 to 24 Gy depending on size.

- No difference in OS (5.7 months vs. 6.5 months).
- OS better with SRS in patients with one met (4.9 months vs. 6.5 months) and RPA Class I.
- Local control at 1 year (71% vs. 82%), KPS better at 6 months, decreased steroid use with addition of SRS.

*SRS alone versus SRS + WBRT*

### JROSG 99-1 (Aoyama, *JAMA* 2006; DOI: 10.1001/jama.295.21.2483)

132 patients. 1 to 4 mets; Lesions <3 cm; RPA II 85%; randomized to SRS alone (18–25 Gy) versus WBRT (30 Gy in 10 fx) + SRS (dose reduced by 30%); 1° end point: OS

- No difference in OS (8 months vs. 7.5 months), neurologic death (19% vs. 23%), or neurocognitive measures (MMSE).

- Addition of WBRT showed better local control (73% vs. 89%), distant brain control (36% vs. 58%), and less need for salvage treatments.

### MD Anderson (Chang, *Lancet Oncol* 2009; DOI: 10.1016/S1470-2045(09)70263-3)

58 patients. 1 to 3 mets (57% single); RPA II 83%; randomized to SRS alone (15–24 Gy) versus SRS first followed by WBRT (30 Gy in 12 fx); 1° end point: assessing neurocognitive function using HVLT-R recall test at 4 months.

- Worse neurocognitive decline in learning and memory with addition of WBRT at 4 months (24% vs. 52%).
- Better LC (67% vs. 100%), distant control (27% vs. 73%), and less salvage treatment with WBRT (11% vs. 90%).
- OS better with SRS alone (15.2 months vs. 5.7 months).

### EORTC 22952-26001 (Kocher, *J Clin Oncol* 2011; DOI: 10.1200/JCO.2010.30.1655 and Soffietti, *J Clin Oncol* 2013; DOI: 10.1200/JCO.2011.41.0639)

359 patients. 1 to 3 mets (<3.5 cm); surgery/SRS randomized to WBRT (30 Gy in 10 fx) or observation; 1° end point: time to WHO PS > 2

- median time to WHO PS > 2 was 10 months after observation versus 9.5 months after WBRT.
- No change in OS 10.9 versus 10.7 months.
- Addition of WBRT improved local relapse (surgery: 59%–27%, radiosurgery: 31%–19%), distant relapse (surgery: 42%–23%, radiosurgery: 48%–33%), less salvage therapy, and reduced neurological death (44% vs. 28%).
- Patients reported better health-related quality of life outcomes (HRQOL) in observation arm compared to WBRT arm.

### Alliance N0574 (Brown, *ASCO* 2015; http://meeting.ascopubs.org/cgi/content/abstract/33/18_suppl/LBA4?sid=7e04d919-8588-4d7f-817f-94b03482f73c)

213 patients. 1 to 3 mets, <3 cm; randomized patients to SRS alone versus SRS + WBRT. 1° end point: cognitive progression (CP) defined as decline >1 SD from baseline in any of the 6 cognitive tests at 3 months

- CP at 3 months was more frequent after WBRT + SRS versus SRS alone 88% versus 62%. More deterioration in the WBRT arm in immediate recall, delayed recall, and verbal fluency.
- WBRT arm improved 1 year local control (51% vs. 85%)
- No change in OS with addition of WBRT (10.1 months vs. 7.5 months).

*Multiple Brain Mets*
*SRS alone*

### JLGK0901 (Yamamoto, *Lancet Oncol* 2014; DOI: 10.1016/S1470-2045(14)70061-0)

1,194 patients. Prospective observational study treated with SRS alone (20–22 Gy) 1 to 10 mets, <3 cm; (largest lesion <10 mL, total cumulative volume ≤15 mL); $1°$ end point: OS, noninferiority margin for the comparison of patients w/2 to 4 brain metastases w/5 to 10 brain mets was set as HR 1.3.

- OS same for 5 to 10 mets versus 2 to 4 mets (10.8 months), HR 1.18.
- SRS may be reasonable to treat in up to 10 mets.

# 2: GLIOBLASTOMA MULTIFORME

*Ahmet Tunceroğlu, MD, PhD*
*Sabin B. Motwani, MD*

## WORKUP

### All Cases

- H&P (make note of age, performance status, neuro deficits)
- CT head and MRI brain (T1 + contrast: thick, irregular enhancing margins, central necrotic core. T2: surrounded by vasogenic edema).

### Considerations

Methylation of the promoter for $O^6$-methylguanine-DNA methyltransferase (MGMT), a DNA repair enzyme. Methylation increases sensitivity to temozolomide (TMZ).

## TREATMENT RECOMMENDATIONS BY AGE AND KPS

| | |
|---|---|
| Age < 70, KPS ≥ 60 | Maximum safe resection → standard fractionation chemoRT → adjuvant chemo |
| Age < 70, KPS < 60 | Standard RT<br>OR hypofx RT<br>OR short 1 week RT course<br>OR chemo alone (if MGMT methylated)<br>OR palliative care |
| Age > 70, KPS ≥ 60 | Maximum safe resection → standard fractionation chemoRT → adjuvant chemo<br>OR hypofx chemoRT → adjuvant chemo<br>OR chemo alone (if MGMT methylated) |
| Age > 70, KPS < 60 | Hypofx RT alone<br>OR short 1-week RT course<br>OR chemo alone (if MGMT methylated)<br>OR palliative care |

Chemo = temozolomide.
In definitively managed cases, perform max safe resection before RT + TMZ for surgical candidates.

## TECHNICAL CONSIDERATIONS

### Simulation

Simulate and treat with aquaplast mask. Obtain pre-op and post-op T1 post contrast and T2 FLAIR MRI images, fuse to CT if no MRI sim.

**Dose Prescription**

*RT Alone*
- Hypofx RT: 40 Gy in 15 fx
- Hypofx RT: 34 Gy in 10 fx
- Short 1-week course: 25 Gy in 5 fx

*Definitive ChemoRT*
- 46 Gy in delivered to microscopic disease (PTV 46) with boost to 60 Gy delivered to gross disease (PTV 60) in 2 Gy/fx.

*TMZ Dose*
- Concurrent: 75 mg/m$^2$/d × **7 d/wk**
- Adjuvant: 150 mg/m$^2$/d × **5 d/month** × 6 months

**Target Delineation**
- Treat initial PTV 46 then cone down to PTV 60

*Initial Fields*
- GTV 46 = T1 enhancement + T2 FLAIR signal + tumor bed
- CTV 46 = GTV 46 + 2 cm, crop at natural barriers (dura, ventricles, falx, tentorium cerebelli)
- PTV 46 = CTV 46 + 0.3 to 0.5 cm

*Cone Down*
- GTV 60 = T1 enhancement + tumor bed
- CTV 60 = GTV 60 + 2 cm
- PTV 60 = CTV 60 + 0.3 to 0.5 cm

*Hypofx RT Target Delineation*
- GTV 40 = T1 enhancement + tumor bed
- CTV 40 = GTV 40 + 2 cm
- PTV 40 = CTV 40 + 0.3 to 0.5 cm

*ASTRO 2015 Recommendations*
- One-phase planning may be utilized in lieu of two-phase RT (46 Gy + boost to 60 Gy).
  - GTV 60 = T1 enhancement + tumor bed
  - CTV 60 = GTV 60 + 2 to 3 cm
  - PTV 60 = CTV 60 + 0.5 to 0.7 cm

**Treatment Planning**

- Intensity-modulated radiation therapy (IMRT) using 6-MV photons
- Multiple beams and/or arcs, consider some noncoplanar beams/arcs
- Avoid beam entrance/exit through mouth, lenses

## FOLLOW UP

If asymptomatic: MRI brain and H&P 2 to 6 weeks after RT, then q2 to 4 months for 2 to 3 years.

Pseudoprogression: Radiation induced necrosis. Occurs in 20% to 30% of patients. Can be very difficult to differentiate from disease recurrence/progression on MRI.

- RANO proposed criteria (Wen et al., *J Clin Oncol* 2010; DOI: 10.1200/JCO.2009.26.3541).
  - If <12 weeks post chemoRT: new enhancement must be out of high-dose RT field (80% isodose line) or must have histologic evidence of recurrence.
  - If >12 weeks post chemoRT: new enhancement out of RT field, ≥25% increase in sum of product of diameters, or clinical deterioration.

Consider obtaining magnetic resonance (MR) spectroscopy or MR perfusion study, especially if within 3 months of completing RT.

## SELECTED STUDIES

### EORTC 26981/22981/NCIC "Stupp Trial" (Stupp, *NEJM* 2005; DOI: 10.1056/NEJMoa043330)

573 patients (84% s/p resection) randomized to 60 Gy RT versus RT + concurrent + adjuvant TMZ.

- Median overall survival (OS) improved with RT + TMZ (14.6 months) versus RT (12.1 months).
- In MGMT-methylated patients, median OS improved from 15.3 months with RT alone, compared to 21.7 months with RT + TMZ.
- Long-term update (*Lancet Oncology* 2009; DOI: 10.1016/S1470-2045(09)70172-X) showed improved 5-year OS with RT + TMZ (9.8%) versus RT (1.9%).
- MGMT methylation status highest predictor both of survival with RT alone and with TMZ.

### Nordic Trial (Malmstrom, *Lancet Oncology* 2012; DOI: 10.1016/S1470-2045(12)70265-6)

342 patients, >60-year old randomized to standard RT 60 Gy in 30 fx versus hypofx RT 34 Gy/10 fx versus 6 1-month cycles TMZ 200 mg/m$^2$/d.

- Median OS similar between TMZ (8.4 months) versus hypofx RT (7.4 months).
- For patients >70-year old, improved median OS compared to standard RT with TMZ (HR 0.35) and hypofx RT (0.59).

### Roa Study (Roa, *J Clin Oncol* 2004; DOI: 10.1200/JCO.2004.06.082)

100 patients, ≥60-year old, s/p resection, randomized to standard RT 60 Gy in 30 fx versus hypofx RT 40 Gy in 15 fx.

- Median OS similar between standard RT (5.1 months) versus hypofx RT (5.6 months).
- More patients in standard arm required increase in post-treatment steroids (49% vs. 23%).

### Italian Trial (Minniti, *Int J Radiat Oncol Biol Phys* 2015; DOI: 10.1016/j.ijrobp.2014.09.013)

Retrospective review of 243 patients, ≥65-year old, comparing standard RT 60 Gy in 30 fx + TMZ versus hypofx RT 40 Gy in 15 fx + TMZ. Median OS similar between standard RT (12 months) versus hypofx RT (12.5 months).

### IAEA Study (Roa *J Clin Oncol* 2015; DOI: 10.3892/mco.2015.515)

Prospectively randomized 98 elderly (≥65 years) and/or frail (KPS 50–70) patients to hypofx RT 40 Gy in 5 fx over 3 weeks versus short-course RT 25 Gy/5 fx over 1 week. No significant difference between short-course RT and standard hypofx RT for median OS (7.9 months vs. 6.9 months), PFS (4.2 months vs. 4.2 months), and quality of life.

### EF-14 NovoTTF Study (Stupp JAMA 2015; DOI: 10.1001/jama.2015.16669)

Randomized patients to tumor treating fields (TTF) + Temodar versus Temodar alone after chemoradiation. Interim analysis of 210 patients. OS greater for TTF patients (20.5 months vs.

15.6 months). PFS improved as well (7.1 months vs. 4 months). TTF was delivered continuously (>18 hr/d) via four transducer arrays placed on the shaved scalp and connected to a portable medical device. Concerns about trial design. Confirmatory trials underway.

### NRG BN001 (Currently Ongoing)

Phase II dose escalation study with a target of 576 patients randomized to either standard RT of 46 Gy with boost to 60 Gy versus dose-painted IMRT or proton RT delivering 50 Gy with boost to 75 Gy. Both arms will receive concurrent and adjuvant TMZ.

### NCT01894061 (Currently Ongoing)

Prospective Phase II trial assessing benefit of adding bevacizumab (VEGF inhibitor) to NovoTTF-100A, a device worn on the scalp that creates electric fields to stunt tumor cell growth.

# 3: LOW-GRADE GLIOMA

*Sabin B. Motwani, MD*

## WORKUP

### All Cases
- H&P (make note of age, performance status, neuro deficits . . . especially hx of seizures)
- CT head and MRI brain w/ and w/o contrast

### Considerations
- 1p19q codeletion
- IDH1 mutation

Risk factors: age >40, astrocytic subtype, size >6 cm, tumor crossing midline, and neuro deficits before surgery (Pignatti et al., *J Clin Oncol* 2002; DOI: 10.1200/JCO.2002.08.121)

## TREATMENT RECOMMENDATIONS BY HISTOLOGIC SUBTYPE

| | |
|---|---|
| Astrocytoma/mixed Astrocytoma/ oligodendroglioma: gross total resection (GTR) or subtotal total resection (STR) and low risk[a] and (1p19q codeletion, ±IDH1+) | Observe (preferred)[b] OR Consider chemotherapy alone (Cat 2B recommendation per National Comprehensive Cancer Network [NCCN]) OR RT |
| Astrocytoma/mixed Astrocytoma/ oligodendroglioma: GTR or STR and low risk[a] and (1p19q noncodeleted, ±IDH1+) | Observe OR RT (preferred) OR Consider chemotherapy alone (Cat 2B recommendation per NCCN) |
| Astrocytoma/mixed Astrocytoma/ oligodendroglioma: GTR or STR and high risk[a] and (±1p19q codeletion, ±IDH1+) | RT → chemo procarbazine, lomustine, vincristine (PCV) OR ChemoRT with temozolomide (TMZ) → chemo (TMZ) |

[a]Low risk is 0 to 2 risk factors and high risk is defined as ≥3 Pignatti risk factors.
[b]Radiation preferred if seizures from the tumor.

## TECHNICAL CONSIDERATIONS

### Simulation
Simulate and treat with aquaplast mask. Obtain post-op T1 post and T2 FLAIR MRI images. MRI sim or fuse MRI images to CT sim images.

### Dose Prescription
- Low risk: RT alone
- 45 to 54 Gy in 1.8 to 2.0 Gy/fx
- High risk: RT + chemo
- 54 Gy in 1.8 Gy/fx followed by six cycles PCV q6 weeks
- OR
- 54 Gy in 1.8 Gy/fx with concurrent TMZ → adjuvant TMZ

#### TMZ Dose
- Concurrent: 75 mg/m$^2$/d × **7 d/wk**
- Adjuvant: 150 mg/m$^2$/d × **5 d/month** × 6 months (if tolerates 150 mg/m$^2$ for first cycle, then raise to 200 mg/m$^2$ for subsequent cycles)

### Target Delineation
- GTV = T1 enhancement + T2 FLAIR signal + tumor bed
- CTV = GTV + 1.5 cm, crop at natural barriers (dura, ventricles, falx, tentorium cerebelli)
- PTV = CTV + 0.3 to 0.5 cm

### Treatment Planning
- Intensity-modulated radiation therapy with 6-MV photons
- Avoid beam entrance/exit through mouth or lenses
- Multiple beams and/or arcs, consider some noncoplanar beams/arcs

## FOLLOW UP
- If asymptomatic: MRI brain and H&P 2 to 6 weeks after RT and then q3 to 6 months for 5 years, then annually
- Pseudoprogression: radiation-induced necrosis. Can occur in 20% to 30% of patients and can be very difficult to differentiate from disease recurrence/progression on MRI.
- RANO proposed criteria (Wen et al., *J Clin Oncol* 2010; DOI: 10.1200/JCO.2009.26.3541)
  - If <12 weeks post chemoRT: new enhancement must be out of high-dose RT field (80% isodose line) or must have histologic evidence of recurrence.

- If >12 weeks post chemoRT: new enhancement out of RT field, ≥25% increase in sum of product of diameters, or clinical deterioration.

Consider obtaining MR spectroscopy, especially if within 3 months of completing RT.

## SELECTED STUDIES

### Dose

### EORTC 22844 "Believers trial" (Karim, *Int J Radiat Oncol Biol Phys* 1996; DOI: 10.1016/S0360-3016(96)00352-5)
343 patients (60% astrocytoma/22% oligo/9% mixed oligo), randomized to 45 Gy versus 59.4 Gy after surgery (25% GTR, 30% STR, and 45% biopsy)

- No difference in overall survival (OS) (58% vs. 59%) or PFS (47% vs. 50%) at 5 years.
- Age, extent of resection, histology, T-stage, and neurological status were found to be prognostic factors.

### Intergroup NCCTG/RTOG/ECOG (Shaw, *J Clin Oncol* 2002; DOI: 10.1200/JCO.2002.09.126)
203 patients (32% astrocytoma/68% oligo + mixed oligo), randomized to 50.4 Gy versus 64.8 Gy after surgery (14% GTR, 35% STR, and 51% biopsy)

- No significant difference in OS (72% low dose vs. 64% high dose) at 5 years.
- Two-year incidence of Grade 3 to 5 RT neurotoxicity (2.5% low dose vs. 5% high dose).
- Favorable prognostic factors are <40 years, tumor size < 5 cm, oligo histology, and GTR.

### Timing of RT

### EORTC 22845 "Non-believers trial" (van den Bent, *Lancet* 2005; DOI: 10.1016/S0140-6736(05)67070-5)
311 patients (62% astrocytoma/25% oligo/10% oligoastro) randomized after surgery (43% GTR, 20% STR, 37% biopsy) to early radiotherapy (54 Gy) versus delayed radiotherapy at time of progression

- Early RT improved median PFS 5.3 years versus 3.4 years and 5 year PFS 55% versus 35%.

- No difference in 5-year OS 68% versus 66%.
- Better control of seizures at 1 year with early RT (25% vs. 41%).
- No difference in rate of malignant transformation to higher grade tumors (~70%).
- Caveats: tumor planning off CT; central path showed 25% were high-grade tumors, 35% of patients in delayed RT never got RT.

### Role of Chemotherapy

### RTOG 9802 (Shaw *J Clin Oncol* 2012; DOI: 10.1200/JCO.2011.35.8598, Buckner *N Engl J Med* 2016; DOI: 10.1056/NEJMoa1500925)

362 patients: Low-risk low-grade glioma (LGG) (age <40 and GTR 111 patients): observation alone

- Low risk: 5-year OS 94%; PFS 50%.
  - High-risk LGG (age >40 or STR/bx 251 patients): randomized to RT alone (54 Gy/30 fx) versus RT + six cycles of adjuvant PCV); Median F/u: 11.9 years
- High-risk: median PFS 10.4 years with the addition of PCV versus 4 years with radiation alone (SS).
- Median OS: 13.3 years with addition of chemo versus 7.8 years RT alone (SS).
- OS: 60% with chemo versus 40% RT alone at 10 years.

### RTOG 0424 (Fisher, *Int J Radiat Oncol Biol Phys* 2015; DOI: 10.1016/j.ijrobp.2014.11.012)

Phase II study, 129 patients with LGG with three or more risk factors (Pignatti) treated with RT (54 Gy/30 fx) and concurrent and adjuvant TMZ

- 3-year OS 73% and is higher than historical controls (54%).

# 4: HIGH-GRADE GLIOMA

*Ahmet Tunceroğlu, MD, PhD*
*Sabin B. Motwani, MD*

## WORKUP

### All Cases

- H&P (make note of age, performance status, neuro deficits)
- CT head and MRI brain w/ and w/o contrast (variable, but generally some enhancement on T1 + contrast, no frank central necrosis)

### Considerations

- 1p19q codeletion (increases sensitivity to procarbazine, lomustine, vincristine [PCV] chemo)
- Isocitrate dehydrogenase (IDH) mutation

## TREATMENT RECOMMENDATIONS BY HISTOLOGIC SUBTYPE

| | |
|---|---|
| 1p19q codeleted or IDH1 mutated<br>Anaplastic oligodendroglioma (AO)<br>Anaplastic oligoastrocytoma (AOA)<br>Anaplastic astrocytoma (AA) | Maximum safe resection → chemo with PCV → standard fractionation RT<br>OR maximum safe resection → standard fractionation RT → chemo (PCV)<br>OR maximum safe resection → chemoRT with temozolomide (TMZ) → adjuvant chemo (TMZ) |
| 1p19q uni- or noncodeleted, and IDH1 wild type<br>AO<br>AOA<br>AA | Maximum safe resection → chemoRT with TMZ → chemo (TMZ) |
| Poor performance status (KPS < 60) | Standard fractionation RT<br>OR hypofx (preferred) external beam radiation therapy<br>OR palliative care |

## TECHNICAL CONSIDERATIONS

### Simulation

Simulate and treat with aquaplast mask. Obtain pre- and post-op T1 post contrast and T2 FLAIR MRI, fuse to CT if no MRI sim.

## Dose Prescription

*Definitive RT*
- 59.4 Gy in 33 fx or 60 Gy in 30 fx

*Hypofractionated RT*
- 40 Gy in 15 fx

*Post-Op ChemoRT*
- 59.4 Gy in 33 fx (cone down after 50.4 Gy) followed by six cycles PCV q6 weeks
- Or four cycles PCV q6 weeks followed by 59.4 Gy in 33 fx (cone down after 50.4 Gy)
- Or 60 Gy in 30 fx (cone down after 46 Gy) with concurrent and adjuvant TMZ

*TMZ Dose*
- Concurrent: 75 mg/m$^2$/d × **7 d/wk**
- Adjuvant: 150 mg/m$^2$/d × **5 d/month** × 6 months (if tolerates 150 mg/m$^2$ for first cycle, then raise to 200 mg/m$^2$ for subsequent cycles)

## Target Delineation

Treat initial PTV 50.4 (or PTV 46) then cone down to PTV 59.4 (or PTV 60)

*Initial Fields*
- GTV 50.4 = T1 enhancement + T2 FLAIR signal + tumor bed
- CTV 50.4 = GTV 50.4 + 2 cm, crop at natural barriers (dura, ventricles, falx, tentorium cerebelli)
- PTV 50.4 = CTV 50.4 + 0.3 to 0.5 cm

*Cone Down*
- GTV 59.4 = T1 enhancement + tumor bed
- CTV 59.4 = GTV 59.4 + 1 to 1.5 cm
- PTV 59.4 = CTV 59.4 + 0.3 to 0.5 cm

*Hypofx RT Target Delineation*
- GTV 40 = T1 enhancement + tumor bed
- CTV 40 = GTV 40 + 2 cm
- PTV 40 = CTV 40 + 0.3 to 0.5 cm

**Treatment Planning**

- Intensity-modulated radiation therapy with 6-MV photons
- Multiple beams and/or arcs, consider some noncoplanar beams/arcs
- Avoid beam entrance/exit through mouth, lenses

## FOLLOW UP

If asymptomatic: MRI brain and H&P 2 to 6 weeks after RT, then q2 to 4 months for 2 to 3 years

Pseudoprogression: Radiation-induced necrosis. Can occur in 20% to 30% of patients and can be very difficult to differentiate from disease recurrence/progression on MRI.

- RANO proposed criteria (Wen et al., *J Clin Oncol* 2010; DOI: 10.1200/JCO.2009.26.3541)
    - If <12 weeks post chemoRT: new enhancement must be out of high-dose RT field (80% isodose line) or must have histologic evidence of recurrence.
    - If >12 weeks post chemoRT: new enhancement out of RT field, ≥25% increase in sum of product of diameters, or clinical deterioration.

Consider obtaining magnetic resonance spectroscopy, especially if within 3 months of completing RT.

## SELECTED STUDIES

### RTOG 9402 (Cairncross, *J Clin Oncol* 2006; DOI: 10.1200/JCO.2005.04.3414)

289 patients (AOA and AO), 88% s/p resection, randomized to 59.4 Gy RT alone versus four cycles PCV followed by 59.4 Gy RT.

- PCV improved progression-free survival (PFS) (2.6 vs. 1.7 years) but not 3-year overall survival (OS).
- Patients with 1p19q codeletion had longer survival compared to noncodeleted (>7 years vs. 2.8 years).
- Long-term update (Cairncross 2013) showed improved OS in codeleted patients with sequential PCV + RT (14.7 years) versus RT alone (7.3 years). No benefit of PCV for noncodeleted patients.

### RTOG 9402 Subgroup Analysis (Cairncross *J Clin Oncol* 2014; DOI: 10.1200/JCO.2013.49.3726)

Retrospective analysis of patient population from RTOG 9402 to evaluate for potential survival advantage of IDH mutation in the context of PCV treatment.

- OS improved with sequential PCV > RT versus RT alone in patients with IDH mutation both in the background of 1p19q codeletion (14.7 years vs. 6.8 years) and in noncodeleted patients (5.5 years vs. 3.3 years).

### EORTC 26951 (Van Den Bent, *J Clin Oncol* 2013; DOI: 10.1200/JCO.2012.43.2229)

368 patients (AO) randomized to 59.4 Gy RT alone versus 59.4 Gy RT followed by six cycles PCV.

- Median OS improved with sequential RT > PCV (42.3 months) versus RT (30.6 months).
- Even greater benefit in 1p19q codeleted patients with sequential RT > PCV versus RT alone for PFS (150 months vs. 50 months) and OS (not reached vs. 112 months).

### NOA-04 Trial (Wick, *J Clin Oncol* 2009; DOI: 10.1200/JCO.2009.23.6497)

318 patients (AO, AOA, and AA), 80% s/p resection, randomized to 60 Gy RT versus chemo (PCV or TMZ). Patients switched arms if unacceptable toxicity or disease progression.

- Time to treatment failure, PFS, or OS did not differ based on whether initial treatment was RT or chemo.

### CODEL Trial (Currently Ongoing)

Initially to evaluate role of TMZ in 1p19q codeleted patients.

- Patients randomized to RT + PCV versus RT + TMZ versus TMZ alone (3-arm study).
- As of 08/15, randomization is now . . . RT + PCV versus RT + TMZ concurrent/adjuvant TMZ (2-arm study). TMZ-alone arm closed due interim data revealing TMZ-alone treated patients would be unlikely to have equivalent or superior survival outcome to patients treated on the two RT containing arms. TMZ arm was also underpowered.

**CATNON Trial (Reported ASCO 2016)**

To evaluate role of TMZ in patients without 1p19q codeletion.

- Patients randomized to RT alone versus RT + concurrent TMZ versus RT + adjuvant TMZ versus RT + concurrent + adjuvant TMZ (4-arm study).

- Adjuvant TMZ improved PFS as well as OS compared to regimens without adjuvant TMZ (5 year OS 56% vs. 44%).

- Concurrent TMZ (vs. RT alone) results still pending.

# 5: MENINGIOMA

*Trevor Bledsoe, MD*
*Sameer Nath, MD*

## WORKUP

- Many cases are asymptomatic and discovered incidentally on imaging.
- H&P (headaches, seizures, visual changes, hearing loss, mental status changes, extremity weakness) including a thorough neurological exam.
- MRI with contrast for diagnosis and treatment planning.

## MENINGIOMA SUBTYPES

| WHO Grade I (benign) | • <4 mitoses per 10 high powered field (HPF).<br>• Meningothelial, fibrous (fibroblastic), transitional (mixed), psammomatous, angiomatous, microcystic, secretory, lympoplasmacyte-rich, and metaplastic. |
|---|---|
| WHO Grade II (atypical) | • ≥4 mitoses per 10 HPF.<br>• Brain invasion.<br>• Three or more of the following.<br>  • Sheeting architecture.<br>  • Hypercellularity.<br>  • Prominent nucleoli.<br>  • Small cells with high nuclear-to-cytoplasmic ratio.<br>  • Foci of spontaneous necrosis.<br>• Atypical, clear cell (intracranial), and choroid. |
| WHO Grade III (anaplastic/malignant) | • >20 per 10 HPF.<br>• Papillary, rhabdoid, anaplastic (malignant). |

## SIMPSON GRADING SYSTEM FOR SURGICAL RESECTION

| Grade I | Complete resection, including resection of dural attachment and abnormal bone |
|---|---|
| Grade II | Complete resection, including coagulation of dural attachment |

(continued)

(*continued*)

| Grade III | Complete resection without resection or coagulation of dural attachment |
| Grade IV | Subtotal resection |
| Grade V | Decompression or biopsy only |

## TREATMENT RECOMMENDATIONS BY SUBTYPE

| WHO Grade I | <ul><li>Small (<3 cm) incidentally found, asymptomatic meningiomas can be observed with serial imaging, reserving treatment for tumor progression.</li><li>Surgical resection favored if accessible.</li><li>Definitive RT favored if potential neurologic consequences from surgery.</li><li>Consider adjuvant RT for subtotal resection.</li><li>SRS: reasonable alternative for small (<3 to 4 cm) tumors.</li></ul> |
|---|---|
| WHO Grade II | <ul><li>Surgical resection if accessible.</li><li>Adjuvant RT is controversial following Simpson Grade I resection of WHO Grade II meningioma, but adjuvant RT is generally otherwise recommended.</li><li>Definitive RT if potential neurologic consequences from surgery.</li></ul> |
| WHO Grade III | <ul><li>Surgical resection followed by adjuvant RT for all cases.</li><li>Definitive RT if potential neurologic consequences from surgery.</li></ul> |

## TECHNICAL CONSIDERATIONS

### Simulation

- Supine; head and neck in a neutral position. Immobilize using a fixed, noninvasive, stereotactic system.
- Simulation CT scan with thin cuts should be performed with contrast when possible and fused with MRI imaging for treatment planning.

**Dose Prescription**
- WHO Grade I
  - 45 to 54 Gy in 25 to 30 fx
  - SRS: 12 to 16 Gy
- WHO Grade II
  - 54 to 60 Gy in 30 fx
- WHO Grade III
  - 59.4 Gy in 33 fx or 60 Gy in 30 fx

**Per RTOG 0539**
- Low risk: WHO Grade I meningioma after GTR (Simpson Grades I–III) or STR (Simpson Grades IV–V) → observation.
- Intermediate risk: WHO Grade II after GTR, or recurrent WHO Grade I regardless of extent of resection → 54 Gy in 30 fractions.
- High risk: WHO Grade III of any resection extent; recurrent WHO Grade II; or WHO Grade II subtotally resected → 60 Gy in 30 fractions.

**Target Delineation**
- GTV
  - Definitive cases: enhancing mass on postcontrast T1-weighted MRI.
  - Post-op cases: tumor bed and any residual nodular enhancement on post-op MRI.
  - Dural tail not included in GTV unless nodular enhancement seen.
- CTV
  - WHO Grade I: CTV = GTV.
  - WHO Grade II (per RTOG 0539): CTV = GTV + 1 cm. Expansion can be reduced to 0.5 cm at natural barriers to tumor growth (e.g., skull).
  - WHO Grade III (per RTOG 0539): $CTV_{60}$ = GTV + 1 cm. $CTV_{54}$ = GTV + 2 cm.
- PTV
  - CTV + 0.3 to 0.5 cm depending on localization method and reproducibility.

**Treatment Planning and Delivery**
- Intensity-modulated radiation therapy or volumetric modulated arc therapy.
- ≥6-MV photons.
- Image-guided radiation therapy.

## FOLLOW UP

- MRI at 6 and 12 months following RT, then every 6 to 12 months for 5 years, then every 1 to 3 years. Consider more frequent imaging after treatment for WHO Grade III disease, recurrent disease, or meningiomas treated with chemotherapy.

## SELECTED STUDIES

### RTOG 0539 (Rodgers, *ASTRO* 2015; DOI: 10.1016/j.ijrobp.2015.07.331)

Randomized trial of patients with meningioma allocated to three different treatment strategies by WHO Grades (I–III), recurrence status, and extent of resection. The first report of RTOG-0539 was presented at *ASTRO* 2015. Patients with WHO Grade II disease who underwent a GTR (Simpson Grades I–III) and patients with recurrent WHO Grade I disease who underwent resection of any extent comprised the intermediate-risk group. Patients in the intermediate-risk group experienced a 3-year progression-free survival (PFS) of 96% with minimal acute or late adverse events above Grade II.

### Goldsmith, *J Neurosurg* 1994; DOI: 10.3171/jns.1994.80.2.0195

Retrospective review of 140 patients treated with adjuvant RT after subtotal resection at UCSF from 1967 to 1990. Benign meningiomas treated to a dose >52 Gy had a PFS rate of 93% compared with 65% for those treated to ≤52 Gy.

### Pollock, *Int J Radiat Oncol Biol Phys* 2003; DOI: 10.1016/S0360-3016(02)04356-0

Retrospective review of 198 patients treated with surgical resection ($n = 136$) or radiosurgery ($n = 62$). All patients had a benign meningioma <35 mm in average diameter. Average margin dose was 17.7 Gy. Patients who underwent radiosurgery had 3- and 7-year PFS rate of 100% and 95%, respectively. No significant difference in PFS was seen among patients with Simpson Grade I resection and patients who underwent radiosurgery. Higher PFS rates were seen among those who underwent radiosurgery compared with patients with Simpson Grade II or Grades III to IV resection. Complications occurred in 10% of patients who underwent radiosurgery compared with 22% of patients who underwent surgical resection ($P = .06$).

**Flickinger,** *Int J Radiat Oncol Biol Phys* **2003;**
**DOI: 10.1016/S0360-3016(02)04356-0**

Retrospective review of 219 cases of meningioma diagnosed by imaging criteria treated with radiosurgery to a median marginal tumor dose of 14 Gy. Actuarial tumor control rate was 93% at 5 and 10 years. Rate of any complication was 5% among patients treated between 1991 and 2000.

# 6: PITUITARY TUMORS

*Trevor Bledsoe, MD*
*Sameer Nath, MD*

## WORKUP

- H&P including detailed cranial nerve exam.
- Formal visual field testing.
- Endocrine workup.
- MRI with and without gadolinium contrast; 1-mm slices through pituitary.
- Microadenoma <1 cm; macroadenoma ≥1 cm.

## TREATMENT RECOMMENDATIONS BY TUMOR TYPE

| | |
|---|---|
| Nonfunctioning adenoma | • Consider observation for asymptomatic microadenoma.<br>• Surgical resection (e.g., trans-sphenoidal surgery) for symptomatic tumors or tumors ≥1 cm.<br>• Consider stereotactic radiosurgery (SRS) or external beam radiation therapy (EBRT) after subtotal resection or at time of disease progression.<br>• No established role for medical therapy. |
| Prolactinoma | • Medical therapy with dopamine agonists (e.g., bromocriptine and cabergoline) is first-line treatment.<br>• Surgery reserved for patients who do not tolerate medical therapy or have rapid progression of symptoms.<br>• Consider RT for patients who fail medical and surgical management. |
| Acromegaly | • Surgery is first-line treatment.<br>• Medical therapy used for patients who have failed surgery or cannot undergo surgery. Includes: somatostatin analogs (e.g., octreotide and lanreotide), dopamine agonists, and GH receptor agonists.<br>• Role of RT controversial; typically reserved for patients who fail surgery and medical therapy. |

*(continued)*

| Cushing's disease | <ul><li>Surgery is first-line treatment.</li><li>RT for patients with persistent disease after surgery and patients unable to undergo surgery.</li><li>Medical therapy reserved for patients who do not respond to surgery and/or RT.</li><li>Salvage bilateral adrenalectomy is an option for patients with persistent or recurrent disease.</li></ul> |
|---|---|

## TECHNICAL CONSIDERATIONS

### Simulation

- Supine; head and neck in a neutral position. Immobilize using a fixed, noninvasive, stereotactic system.
- Simulation CT scan with thin cuts should be performed with contrast, when possible, and fused with MRI imaging for treatment planning.

### Dose Prescription

- SRS
  - Nonfunctioning
    - 14 to 16 Gy to the 50% isodose line
  - Functioning
    - 16 to 35 Gy to the 50% isodose line
    - Higher doses as possible while respecting optic chiasm constraint
- EBRT
  - Nonfunctioning, no gross disease
    - 45 to 50.4 Gy in 25 to 28 fx
  - Functioning
    - 50.4 to 54 Gy in 28 to 30 fx
  - Gross disease
    - 54 Gy in 30 fx

### Target Delineation

- GTV = hypointense or isotense mass on postcontrast, T1-weighted MRI
- CTV = GTV
- PTV = 3 to 5 mm depending on localization method and reproducibility. 0 to 1 mm if treating with SRS

## Treatment Planning

- ▤ Consider holding hormonal therapy for several weeks before RT, as tolerated by patient, to increase response to RT.
- ▤ SRS generally favored over EBRT as it is believed to be associated with shorter times to hormone level renormalization. Consider using EBRT for tumors within 3 to 5 mm of the optic pathway, extensive cavernous sinus involvement, or tumors ≥4 cm in size.
- ▤ EBRT
  - ▤ Intensity-modulated radiation therapy or volumetric-modulated arc therapy
  - ▤ ≥6-MV photons
  - ▤ Image-guided radiation therapy

## FOLLOW UP

MRI every 6 months for 1 year, followed by annual imaging.

- ▤ Endocrine testing
- ▤ Visual field testing

## SELECTED STUDIES

### Grant, *World Neurosurg* 2014; DOI: 10.1016/j.wneu.2013.01.127

Retrospective review of 31 patients with persistent functional pituitary adenomas after surgical resection who underwent adjuvant SRS. Patients were treated to 35 Gy to the 50% isodose line. Compared with previously published studies of treatment to 20 to 24 Gy, time to endocrine remission was more rapid (median 18 months vs. 24–144 months) and rate of remission of hypersecretion was higher (70% vs. approximately 50%) among patients treated to 35 Gy.

### Sheehan, *J Neurosurg* 2013; DOI: 10.3171/2013.3.JNS12766

Retrospective review of 512 patients with nonfunctional pituitary adenomas. 94% had surgery and 7% had EBRT before SRS. Tumor control was 93% at last follow up. New or worsened hypopituitarism after SRS seen in 21%. New or progressive cranial nerve deficits seen in 9% of patients. 7% of patients developed new or worsened optic nerve dysfunction.

### Sheehan, *J Neurosurg* 2011; DOI: 10.3171/2010.5.JNS091635

Retrospective review of 418 patients treated at the University of Virginia between 1989 and 2006. Patients were treated with

SRS for persistently functioning adenoma or for radiographic progression of a nonfunctioning adenoma. Median dose was 24 Gy (9–30). Local control was 90%, time to endocrine remission was 49 months. 24% of patients developed new-onset hypopituitarism. Tumor-margin dose was inversely correlated with time to remission. Large adenoma volume, treatment with hormone suppression, and a prior craniotomy were associated with development of hypopituitarism.

**Sheehan,** *J Neurosurg* **2005; DOI: 10.3171/jns.2007.106.6.980**
Review of 35 studies involving 1,621 patients. Local control with radiosurgery was approximately 90%. Risks of hypopituitarism, radiation-induced neoplasia, and cerebral vasculopathy appeared to be lower among patients treated with SRS than those receiving EBRT.

**Kim,** *Int J Radiat Oncol Biol Phys* **2013;**
**DOI: 10.1016/j.ijrobp.2013.06.2057**
Review of 76 patients with pituitary adenomas who underwent fractionated stereotactic radiation therapy. 71% nonfunctioning, 29% functioning. 96% of patients had previous surgery. Median dose 50.4 Gy in 28 fractions. Median follow-up ~7 years. progression-free survival at 7 years was 97% and disease-specific survival was 100% at 7 years. No cases of optic nerve injury or radionecrosis.

# 7: NASOPHARYNX CANCER

*Arti Parekh, MD*
*Ana Kiess, MD, PhD*

## WORKUP

### All Cases

- H&P including complete head and neck exam, cranial nerve exam, and nasopharyngolaryngoscopy
- MRI with contrast of neck and skull base
- CT with contrast of neck and skull base
- Biopsy primary tumor and/or fine-needle aspiration neck node
- Epstein–Barr virus (EBV) testing on biopsy specimen, serum EBV DNA
- Dental, nutrition, speech, and swallow evaluations

### Stages III to IV

- PET/CT or CT chest
- Consider prophylactic percutaneous endoscopic gastrostomy tube for baseline dysphagia, severe weight loss, or advanced primary
- Consider audiogram
- Labs-complete blood count, comprehensive metabolic panel, thyroid-stimulating hormone (TSH)

## TREATMENT RECOMMENDATIONS BY STAGE

| | |
|---|---|
| T1N0 | Definitive RT |
| T2–4 any N | ChemoRT ➔ adjuvant chemo (preferred)<br>OR chemoRT alone |
| M1 | Platinum-based combination chemo<br>Consider chemoRT to primary in select patients with limited distant metastases, small tumor, or symptomatic disease |

ChemoRT = chemoradiation with cisplatin preferred.

## TECHNICAL CONSIDERATIONS

### Simulation

■ Simulate supine with neck extended, immobilize with thermoplastic mask. Consider mouthpiece with tongue depressor. Consider bolus for disease near skin. IV contrast if no contraindications. Fuse diagnostic imaging.

### Dose Prescription

■ Gross disease: 70 Gy in 35 fx or 70.2 Gy 33 fx
■ Intermediate-risk areas: 63 Gy in 35 fx or 59.4 Gy in 33 fx
■ Low-risk area: 56 Gy in 35 fx or 54 Gy in 33 fx

### Target Delineation

■ GTV = gross disease based on exam and imaging
■ CTV70 = GTV + margin for subclinical disease (5 mm in RTOG 0615)
■ **CTV Intermediate Risk**
   ■ Primary: entire nasopharynx, parapharyngeal space, clivus, foramen ovale, sphenoid sinus, posterior 1/3 of maxillary sinuses, posterior 1.3 of nasal cavity, cavernous sinus for advanced T3 to 4
   ■ Neck: bilateral IB-V and RP if bilateral neck involvement. Ipsilateral IB-V and bilateral RP if only ipsilateral neck involvement. IB can be excluded if N0.
■ CTV low risk = II to V nodes in uninvolved sides of the neck
■ PTV = CTV + 3- to 5-mm margin, depending on image guidance

### Treatment Planning

■ 6-MV photons
■ Intensity-modulated radiation therapy (IMRT) preferred, with image guidance if available

## FOLLOW UP

MRI 3 months after definitive RT/chemoradiation (CRT). If suspicion for residual neck disease, consider neck dissection.

If asymptomatic, H&P and nasopharyngolaryngoscopy every 1 to 3 months for year 1, every 2 to 6 months for year 2, every 4 to 8 months for years 3 to 5, then annually. TSH every 6 to 12 months. Consider serum EBV DNA if initially positive. Management of nutrition, dental, speech, swallow, hearing, and smoking cessation as indicated. Chest imaging as indicated for smoking history.

## SELECTED STUDIES

### INT 0099 (Al-Sarraf, *J Clin Oncol* 1998)

147 patients with stages III to IV nasopharyngeal carcinoma (NPC) randomized to RT alone (70 Gy) versus RT (70 Gy) with concurrent cisplatin and adjuvant cisplatin/5FU. Results show 3-year overall survival (OS) 78% versus 47%, progression-free survival 69% versus 24%. Concluded that CRT superior to RT alone for advanced nasopharyngeal cancer.

### RTOG 0225 (Lee, *J Clin Oncol* 2009; DOI: 10.1200/JCO.2008.19.9109)

68 patients with stages I to IVB NPC all treated with IMRT to 70 Gy. If T2b+ or N+, also received concurrent and adjuvant chemo. Outcomes include 2-year OS 80%, LRC 93%, late-grade 3 dysphagia 5%, and xerostomia 3%.

### Singapore SQNP01 (Wee, *J Clin Oncol* 2005)

221 patients with stages II to III randomized to RT alone (70 Gy) versus RT (70 Gy) with concurrent cisplatin and adjuvant cisplatin/5FU. Results show 3-year OS 80% versus 65%, disease-free survival (DFS) 72% versus 53%. Confirmed results of INT 0099 applicable to endemic NPC.

# 8: NASAL CAVITY AND PARANASAL SINUS

*Sarah Nicholas, MD*
*Ana Kiess, MD, PhD*

## WORKUP

### All Cases

- H&P including complete head and neck exam and nasopharyngolaryngoscopy
- Imaging—contrast-enhanced CT or MRI of neck.
- Biopsy of primary tumor
- Dental, nutrition, speech, and swallow evaluations
- MRI of skull base if concern for perineural spread

### Stages III to IV

- PET/CT or CT chest
- Labs-CBC, CMP, thyroid-stimulating hormone (TSH)

## NASAL CAVITY AND ETHMOID SINUS TREATMENT RECOMMENDATIONS BY STAGE

| T1 to 2 | Surgery (preferred) ➜ adjuvant treatment as indicated (see "Post-op" section) OR definitive RT |
| --- | --- |
| T3 to 4a | Surgery (preferred) ➜ adjuvant treatment as indicated (see "Post-op" section) OR definitive chemoRT |
| Post-op all patients | Adjuvant RT OR consider observation for low grade T1N0 with negative margins and central location OR consider adjuvant chemoRT for positive margins or intracranial extension |
| T4b Unresectable Unfit for surgery | Clinical trial (preferred) OR chemoRT OR definitive RT OR palliation with chemo or RT OR supportive care |
| M1 | Palliation with chemo, RT, or surgery OR supportive care |

## MAXILLARY SINUS TREATMENT RECOMMENDATIONS BY STAGE

| | |
|---|---|
| T1 to 4a | Surgery → adjuvant treatment as indicated (see "Post-op" section) |
| Post-op T1 to T2, N0 | Adjuvant RT for adenoid cystic carcinoma, perineural invasion (PNI) or positive margins (consider adjuvant chemoRT for positive margin) |
| Post-op T3 to 4a, N0 | Adjuvant RT for squamous cell carcinoma, undifferentiated tumors, adenoid cystic carcinoma, PNI, positive margins (consider adjuvant chemoRT) |
| Post-op N+ | Adjuvant RT OR consider adjuvant chemoRT for positive margins or ECE |
| T4b Unresectable Unfit for surgery | Clinical trial (preferred) OR chemoRT OR definitive RT OR palliation with chemo or RT OR supportive care |
| M1 | Palliation with chemo, RT, or surgery OR supportive care |

For sinonasal undifferentiated carcinoma, small cell or neuro-endocrine histologies systemic therapy should be part of the treatment.

## TECHNICAL CONSIDERATIONS

### Simulation

Simulate supine with neck extended, immobilize with thermoplastic mask. Consider mouthpiece and/or tongue depressor. Wire scars. Consider bolus for disease near skin. IV contrast if no contraindications. Fuse pre-op imaging.

**Dose Prescription**

*Definitive RT Alone**

- High-risk areas: 66 Gy in 30 fx, or 70 Gy in 35 fx
- Intermediate-risk areas: 60 Gy in 30 fx, or 63 Gy in 35 fx
- Low-risk areas: 54 Gy in 30 fx, or 56 Gy in 35 fx

*Altered fractionation regimens such as concomitant boost or hyperfractionation are also considered.

*Adjuvant RT*

- High-risk areas: 63 Gy in 30 fx, or 66 Gy in 33 fx
- Intermediate-risk areas: 57 to 60 Gy in 30 fx
- Low-risk areas: 54 Gy in 30 fx

*ChemoRT*

- High-risk areas: 70 Gy in 35 fx
- Intermediate-risk areas: 63 Gy in 35 fx
- Low-risk areas: 56 Gy in 35 fx

**Target Delineation**

*Definitive*

- GTV = gross disease based on exam and imaging
- CTV high risk = GTV + margin for subclinical disease (5–10 mm)
- CTV intermediate risk = entire subsite, nerve track(s) to skull base if PNI or adenoid cystic carcinoma, cribriform plate if esthesioneuroblastoma or ethmoid sinus, ipsilateral neck nodes if N+
- CTV low risk: uninvolved nodes at low risk for subclinical disease**
- PTV = CTV + 3- to 5-mm margin, depending on image guidance

*Post-Op*

- CTV high risk = areas of positive margins
- CTV intermediate risk = tumor bed + entire subsite, nerve track(s) to skull base if PNI or adenoid cystic carcinoma, cribriform plate if esthesioneuroblastoma or ethmoid sinus, ipsilateral neck nodes if N+, post-op areas
- CTV low risk: uninvolved nodes at low risk for subclinical disease**
- PTV: CTV + 3- to 5-mm margin, depending on image guidance

\*\*CTV low risk includes elective nodal regions based on disease site and stage. May be omitted for many cases but should be considered for esthesioneuroblastoma, high-grade squamous cell carcinoma, maxillary sinus cancer, or involvement of nasopharynx or oral cavity.

### Treatment Planning
- 6-MV photons
- Intensity-modulated radiation therapy (IMRT) preferred, with image guidance if available
- Prefer starting post-op cases within 6 weeks postsurgery

### FOLLOW UP

- PET/CT 3 months after definitive RT/chemoradiation. If suspicion for residual neck disease, consider neck dissection. After adjuvant RT, posttreatment baseline imaging of head and neck within 6 months.
- If asymptomatic, H&P and nasopharyngolaryngoscopy every 1 to 3 months for year 1, every 2 to 6 months for year 2, every 4 to 8 months for years 3 to 5, then annually. TSH every 6 to 12 months. Management of nutrition, dental, speech, swallow, hearing, and smoking cessation as indicated. Chest imaging as indicated for smoking history.

### SELECTED STUDIES

#### IMRT for Sinonasal (Madani, *Int J Radiat Oncol Biol Phys* 2009; DOI: 10.1016/j.ijrobp.2008.04.037)
Low toxicity with IMRT for 84 patients with sinonasal tumors (75 patients adjuvant RT, 9 patients definitive RT). Five-year local control 71% and disease-free survival 59%.

#### Post-Op RT for Maxillary Sinus (Bristol, *Int J Radiat Oncol Biol Phys* 2007)
Supports elective nodal irradiation for maxillary sinus cancer with squamous or undifferentiated histology. Regional control 64% without nodal irradiation (vs. 93% with nodal irradiation). Also demonstrated decreased grades 3 to 4 complications with improved dose distribution, improved local control with skull base coverage, and improved nodal control with elective neck irradiation for squamous or undifferentiated histology.

# 9: OROPHARYNX CANCER

*Zach Guss, MD, MSc*
*Ana Kiess, MD, PhD*

## WORKUP

### All Cases
- H&P including complete head and neck exam and nasopharyngolaryngoscopy
- Imaging-contrast-enhanced CT or MRI of neck
- Biopsy primary tumor and/or fine-needle aspiration neck node
- Human papilloma virus (HPV) testing on biopsy specimen
- Dental, nutrition, speech, and swallow evaluations

### Stages III to IV
- PET/CT or CT chest
- Consider prophylactic percutaneous endoscopic gastrostomy tube for baseline dysphagia, severe weight loss, or advanced primary
- Consider audiogram
- Labs-complete blood count, comprehensive metabolic panel, thyroid-stimulating hormone (TSH)

## TREATMENT RECOMMENDATIONS BY STAGE

| All stages | Consider clinical trial, especially de-escalation trials for HPV+ |
|---|---|
| T1 to 2, N0 to 1 | RT (consider chemoRT for T2N1) OR surgery |
| T3 to 4a, N0 to 1 | ChemoRT OR surgery → adjuvant treatment as indicated (see "Post-op" section) |
| Any T, N2 to 3 | ChemoRT OR surgery → adjuvant treatment as indicated (see "Post-op" section) |
| Post-op pT3 to 4, multiple positive nodes, level IV to V nodes, Perineural invasion, or lymphovascular invasion | Adjuvant RT |

*(continued)*

*(continued)*

| Post-op positive margins or extracapsular extension (ECE) | Adjuvant chemoRT |
|---|---|
| T4b, any N<br>Unresectable<br>Unfit for surgery | Clinical trial (preferred)<br>OR chemoRT<br>OR chemo > RT<br>OR definitive RT<br>OR palliation with chemo or RT<br>OR supportive care |
| M1 | Palliation with chemo, RT, or surgery<br>OR supportive care |

## TECHNICAL CONSIDERATIONS

### Simulation

Simulate supine with neck extended, immobilize with thermoplastic mask. Consider mouthpiece. Wire scars. Consider bolus for disease near skin. IV contrast if no contraindications. Fuse diagnostic imaging.

### Dose Prescription

*Definitive RT\**
- High-risk areas: 66 Gy in 30 fx, or 70 Gy in 35 fx
- Intermediate-risk areas: 60 Gy in 30 fx or 63 Gy in 35 fx
- Low-risk areas: 54 Gy in 30 fx or 56 Gy in 35 fx

\*Altered fractionation regimens such as concomitant boost or hyperfractionation are also considered

*Adjuvant RT*
- High-risk areas: 63 Gy in 30 fx, or 66 Gy in 33 fx
- Intermediate-risk areas: 60 Gy in 30 fx
- Low-risk areas: 54 Gy in 30 fx

*ChemoRT*
- High-risk areas: 70 Gy in 35 fx
- Intermediate-risk areas: 63 Gy in 35 fx
- Low-risk areas: 56 Gy in 35 fx

### Target Delineation

*Definitive*
- GTV = gross disease based on exam and imaging
- CTV high risk = GTV + margin for subclinical disease (5–10 mm)

- CTV intermediate risk
    - Base of tongue: glossotonsillar sulcus, mucosal margin, pre epiglottic space
    - Tonsil: glossotonsillar sulcus, parapharyngeal space, adjacent palate, pterygoids if advanced
    - Posterior pharyngeal wall: mucosal margin
    - Neck: bilateral IB to V and bilateral retropharyngeal (RP) if bilateral neck involvement. Ipsilateral IB to V and RP if only ipsilateral neck involvement. Include IA if oral cavity involvement.
- CTV low risk = uninvolved contralateral II to IV nodes (can omit contralateral neck if well lateralized, low-volume tonsil cancer)
- PTV = CTV + 3- to 5-mm margin, depending on image guidance

*Post-Op*
- CTV high risk = areas of positive margins or ECE
- CTV intermediate risk
    - Base of tongue: glossotonsillar sulcus, mucosal margin, pre-epiglottic space
    - Tonsil: glossotonsillar sulcus, parapharyngeal space, adjacent palate, pterygoids if advanced
    - Posterior pharyngeal wall: mucosal margin
    - Neck: bilateral IB to V and RP if bilateral neck involvement. Ipsilateral IB to V and RP if only ipsilateral neck involvement. Include IA if oral cavity involvement. Post-op areas
- CTV low risk = uninvolved contralateral II to IV nodes (can omit contralateral neck if well lateralized, low-volume tonsil cancer)
- PTV = CTV + 3- to 5-mm margin, depending on image guidance

**Treatment Planning**
- 6-MV photons
- Intensity-modulated radiation therapy preferred, with image guidance if available
- Prefer starting post-op cases within 6 weeks postsurgery

**FOLLOW UP**

- PET/CT 3 months after definitive RT/chemoradiation. If suspicion for residual neck disease, consider neck dissection. After adjuvant RT, post-treatment baseline imaging of head and neck within 6 months.

▪ If asymptomatic, H&P and nasopharyngolaryngoscopy every 1 to 3 months for year 1, every 2 to 6 months for year 2, every 4 to 8 months for years 3 to 5, then annually. TSH every 6 to 12 months. Management of nutrition, dental, speech, swallow, hearing, and smoking cessation as indicated. Chest imaging as indicated for smoking history.

## SELECTED STUDIES

### Princess Margaret Ipsilateral RT (O'Sullivan, *Int J Radiat Oncol Biol Phys* 2001)

Retrospective series of 228 patients with tonsil primaries who received ipsilateral neck RT. Mean f/u 7 years, primary T1 to T2N0. Contralateral neck failure in 3.5%.

### ACR Appropriateness Criteria for Ipsilateral RT (Yeung, *Head Neck*, 2012; DOI: 10.1002/hed.21993)

Ipsilateral radiation for squamous cell carcinoma of the tonsil appropriateness criteria.

### HPV and Oropharyngeal Cancer (Ang, *N Engl J Med* 2010; DOI: 10.1056/NEJMoa0912217)

Retrospective analysis of RTOG 0129 patients with stages III to IV oropharyngeal cancer. Showed HPV status is a strong independent prognostic factor (3-year overall survival [OS] 82.4% for HPV+ vs. 57.1% for HPV−).

### EORTC 22931 (Bernier, *N Engl J Med* 2004; DOI: 10.1056/NEJMoa032641)

Post-op treatment of 167 patients testing RT versus cisplatin-based chemoRT for stages III to IV head and neck cancer. Significantly improved progression-free survival (PFS) (47% vs. 36%) and OS (53% vs. 40%) in chemoRT arm, similar toxicities. Combined analysis with RTOG data led to ECE or positive margin as indications for post-op chemoRT.

# 10: ORAL CAVITY AND LIP CANCERS

*Colette Shen, MD*
*Ana Kiess, MD, PhD*

## WORKUP

### All Cases
- H&P including complete head and neck exam
- Nasopharyngolaryngoscopy and/or exam under anesthesia as indicated
- Imaging-contrast-enhanced CT or MRI of neck
- Biopsy primary tumor and/or fine-needle aspiration neck node
- Dental, nutrition, speech, and swallow evaluations

### Stages III to IV
- PET/CT or CT chest
- Consider percutaneous endoscopic gastrostomy tube for dysphagia, weight loss, or advanced primary
- Labs-complete blood count, comprehensive metabolic panel, thyroid-stimulating hormone (TSH)

## TREATMENT RECOMMENDATIONS BY STAGE

| T1 to 2, N0 | Surgery (preferred)<br>OR definitive RT |
|---|---|
| T3, N0<br>T1 to 3, N1 to 3<br>T4a, any N | Oral Cavity:<br>Surgery → adjuvant treatment as indicated<br>(see "Post-op" section)<br>Lip<br>Surgery (preferred) → adjuvant treatment as indicated (see "Post-op" section)<br>OR definitive RT or chemoradiotherapy (CRT) |
| Post-op pT3 to 4, multiple positive nodes, levels IV to V nodes, perineural invasion (PNI), or lymphovascular invasion (LVI) | Adjuvant RT |
| Post-op positive margins or extracapsular spread | Adjuvant CRT<br>OR re-resection for positive margins |

(continued)

| T4b, any N<br>Unresectable<br>Unfit for surgery | Clinical trial (preferred)<br>OR chemoRT<br>OR chemo → RT<br>OR definitive RT<br>OR palliation with chemo or RT<br>OR supportive care |
|---|---|
| M1 | Palliation with chemo, RT, or surgery<br>OR supportive care |

Sites include: anterior 2/3 tongue, buccal mucosa, floor of mouth, alveolar ridge, retromolar trigone, hard palate, upper and lower lips.

## TECHNICAL CONSIDERATIONS

### Simulation
Simulate supine with neck extended, immobilize with thermo-plastic mask. Consider mouthpiece and/or tongue depressor. Wire scars and oral commissure. Consider bolus for disease near skin. IV contrast if no contraindications. Fuse pre-op imaging.

### Site-Specific Notes
- Lip: definitive RT preferred for superficial lesions involving most of lower lip. Small lesions may be treated with definitive RT using external beam radiation therapy (EBRT) (electrons or orthovoltage), brachytherapy, or combination.
- Oral tongue and floor of mouth: Small lesions can be treated with EBRT (photons or intraoral cone electron RT), brachytherapy, or combination. Consider tongue depressor. Careful setup due to mobility of tongue.
- Buccal mucosa: displace tongue with mouthpiece; displace/ shield lips and oral commissure if possible.
- Gingiva and hard palate: brachytherapy not recommended due to risk of osteoradionecrosis. Consider tongue depressor.

### Dose Prescription
*Definitive RT\**
- High-risk areas: 66 Gy in 30 fx, or 70 Gy in 35 fx
- Intermediate-risk areas: 60 Gy in 30 fx or 63 Gy in 35 fx
- Low-risk areas: 54 Gy in 30 fx or 56 Gy in 35 fx

\*Altered fractionation regimens such as concomitant boost or hyperfractionation are also considered

*Adjuvant RT*
- High-risk areas: 63 Gy in 30 fx, or 66 Gy in 33 fx
- Intermediate-risk areas: 60 Gy in 30 fx
- Low-risk areas: 54 Gy in 30 fx

*ChemoRT*
- High-risk areas: 70 Gy in 35 fx
- Intermediate-risk areas: 63 Gy in 35 fx
- Low-risk areas: 56 Gy in 35 fx

*Interstitial Brachytherapy*
- Considered in select cases; low-dose rate (LDR) alone 60 to 70 Gy over several days, LDR boost 20 to 35 Gy (with 50 Gy EBRT); high-dose rate (HDR) alone 45 to 60 Gy in 3 to 6 Gy/fraction, HDR boost 21 Gy in 3 Gy/fraction (with 45–50 Gy EBRT)

**Target Delineation**
*Definitive*
- GTV = gross disease based on exam and imaging
- CTV high risk = GTV + margin for subclinical disease (5–10 mm)
- CTV intermediate risk = nodes at high risk for subclinical disease (typically ipsilateral I–IV if N0, I–V if N+)
- CTV low risk: uninvolved nodes at low risk for subclinical disease*
- PTV = CTV + 3- to 5-mm margin, depending on image guidance

*Post-Op*
- CTV high risk = soft tissue/bone invasion, areas of positive margins or extracapsular extension (ECE)
- CTV intermediate risk = pre-op gross disease and tumor bed; nodes at high risk for subclinical disease (typically ipsilateral I–IV if N0, I–V if N+)
- CTV low risk: uninvolved nodes at low risk for subclinical disease*
- PTV: CTV + 3- to 5-mm margin, depending on image guidance

*CTV low risk typically includes contralateral uninvolved nodes based on disease site and stage. Contralateral neck may be omitted for well lateralized cancers of buccal mucosa, retromolar trigone, hard palate, or gingiva

**Treatment Planning**

- 6-MV photons
- Intensity-modulated radiation therapy preferred, with image guidance if available
- Prefer starting post-op cases within 6 weeks postsurgery

## FOLLOW UP

PET/CT 3 months after definitive radiation or chemoradiation. If suspicion for residual neck disease, consider neck dissection. After adjuvant RT, posttreatment baseline imaging of head and neck within 6 months.

If asymptomatic, H&P and nasopharyngolaryngoscopy every 1 to 3 months for year 1, every 2 to 6 months for year 2, every 4 to 8 months for years 3 to 5, then annually. TSH every 6 to 12 months. Management of nutrition, dental, speech, swallow, hearing, and smoking cessation as indicated. Chest imaging as indicated for smoking history.

## SELECTED STUDIES

### EORTC 22931 (Bernier, *N Engl J Med* 2004)

334 patients with operable stage III/IV oral cavity, oropharynx, larynx, and hypopharynx cancer randomized to post-op RT (66 Gy) versus post-op chemoRT (66 Gy + cisplatin × 3c). ChemoRT improved 5-year progression-free survival (47% vs. 36%), overall survival (OS) (53% vs. 40%), and locoregional control rate (LRC) (82% vs. 69%), but had increased grades 3 to 4 toxicity (41% vs. 21%).

### RTOG 9501 (Cooper, *N Engl J Med* 2004 and *Int J Radiat Oncol Biol Phys* 2012; DOI: 10.1016/j.ijrobp.2012.05.008)

459 patients with operable cancer of the oral cavity, oropharynx, larynx, or hypopharynx with ≥2 involved lymph nodes, nodal ECE, or + margin randomized to post-op RT (60–66 Gy) versus post-op chemoRT (60–66 Gy + cisplatin × 3c). ChemoRT improved 2-year disease-free survival (DFS) and LRC but not OS and increased grades 3 to 4 toxicity. 10-year update: no differences in DFS, OS, LRC; but subset analysis of patients with + margins or ECE showed improved LRC (79% vs. 67%) and DFS (18% vs. 12%).

### Combined Analysis of EORTC 22931 and RTOG 9501 (Bernier, *Head Neck* 2005)

ChemoRT improved DFS and LRC for ECE and/or + margins, but provided only trend for improvements in stages III to IV, PNI, LVI, and/or enlarged levels IV to V nodes. Patients with ≥2 + nodes without ECE as their only risk factor did not benefit from chemo.

### Post-Op RT Risk Features and Time Factors (Ang, *Int J Radiat Oncol Biol Phys* 2001)

213 patients with operable cancer of the oral cavity, oropharynx, larynx, or hypopharynx stratified for adjuvant treatment according to risk factors: ECE >1 nodal group, ≥2 LN+, >3 cm LN, oral cavity, +margins, PNI 5-year LRC for low-risk patients 90% (with no risk factors, no RT), intermediate-risk patients 94% (with one risk factor, RT 58 Gy), and high-risk patients 68% (with 2+ risk factors or ECE, RT 65 Gy conventional/accelerated). Surgery-RT interval >6 weeks associated with decreased LRC.

# 11: MAJOR SALIVARY GLAND TUMORS

*Adam Ferro, MD, MS*
*Ana Kiess, MD, PhD*

## WORKUP

### All Cases
- H&P including complete head and neck exam and cranial nerve exam
- Imaging—contrast-enhanced CT and MRI of neck
- Fine-needle aspiration (FNA) of primary tumor
- Dental and nutrition evaluations prior to radiation

### Stages III to IV
- PET/CT or CT chest
- MRI of skull base if concern for perineural spread

## TREATMENT RECOMMENDATIONS BY STAGE

| | |
|---|---|
| Benign | Surgery. Consider adjuvant RT for recurrent multifocal pleomorphic adenoma. |
| cT1–T4a | Surgery → adjuvant treatment as indicated (see "Post-op" section) |
| Post-op pT1–T2 | Consider adjuvant RT for int/high grade, adenoid cystic histology, tumor spillage, or perineural invasion (PNI) |
| Post-op pT3–T4 | Adjuvant RT for int/high grade, adenoid cystic histology, close/positive margins, PNI, nodal metastases, or LVI<br>OR consider adjuvant chemoRT for positive margins or ECE |
| Gross residual disease T4b<br>Unresectable<br>Unfit for surgery | Definitive RT<br>OR chemoRT<br>OR palliation with chemo or RT<br>OR supportive care |
| M1 | Palliation with chemo, RT, or surgery<br>OR supportive care |

## TECHNICAL CONSIDERATIONS

### Simulation

Simulate supine with neck extended, immobilize with thermoplastic mask. Consider mouthpiece. Wire scars. Consider bolus for disease near skin. Intravenous (IV) contrast if no contraindications. Fuse pre-op imaging.

### Dose Prescription

*Definitive RT*

- High-risk areas: 66 Gy in 30 to 33 fx or 70 Gy in 35 fx
- Intermediate-risk areas: 60 Gy in 30 fx, or 63 Gy in 35 fx
- Low-risk areas: 54 Gy in 30 fx, or 56 Gy in 35 fx

*Adjuvant RT*

- High-risk areas: 63 Gy in 30 fx or 66 Gy in 33 fx
- Intermediate-risk areas: 60 Gy in 30 fx
- Low-risk areas: 54 Gy in 30 fx

*ChemoRT*

- High-risk areas: 70 Gy in 35 fx
- Intermediate-risk areas: 63 Gy in 35 fx
- Low-risk areas: 56 Gy in 35 fx

### Target Delineation

*Definitive*

- GTV = gross disease based on exam and imaging
- Clinical target volume (CTV) high risk = GTV + margin for subclinical disease (5–10 mm)
- CTV intermediate risk:
  - Parotid: entire parotid, facial nerve track if PNI, or adenoid cystic carcinoma
  - Submandibular: entire submandibular, lingual or hypoglossal nerve track if PNI, or adenoid cystic carcinoma
  - Neck: ipsilateral IB-V if node involvement
  - CTV low risk = ipsilateral IB-III if node negative (may omit neck in adenoid cystic or low-grade histologies)
  - PTV = CTV + 3- to 5-mm margin, depending on image guidance

*Post-Op*
- CTV high risk = areas of positive margins or ECE
- CTV intermediate risk:
    - Parotid: entire parotid bed, facial nerve track if PNI, or adenoid cystic carcinoma
    - Submandibular: entire submandibular bed, lingual or hypoglossal nerve track if PNI, or adenoid cystic carcinoma
    - Neck: ipsilateral IB-V if node involvement
    - Post-op areas
- CTV low risk = ipsilateral IB-III if node negative (may omit neck in ACC or low-grade histologies)
- PTV = CTV + 3- to 5-mm margin, depending on image guidance

**Treatment Planning**
- 6-MV photons
- Intensity-modulated radiation therapy (IMRT) preferred, with image guidance if available
- Prefer starting post-op cases within 6-weeks postsurgery

**FOLLOW UP**

Posttreatment baseline imaging of head and neck within 6 months after adjuvant RT. If asymptomatic, H&P every 1 to 3 months for year 1, every 2 to 6 months for year 2, every 4 to 8 months for years 3 to 5, then annually. Thyroid screening every 6 to 12 months. Management of nutrition, dental, speech, swallow, hearing, and smoking cessation as indicated. Chest imaging as indicated for smoking history.

**SELECTED STUDIES**

**UCSF Risk Factors (Chen, *Int J Radiat Oncol Biol Phys* 2007)**
Retrospective study of 207 patients with major salivary carcinomas treated with surgery without post-op radiotherapy. Five- and 10-year local/regional control were 86% and 74%, respectively. Independent predictors of local/regional recurrence were pathologic lymph node metastasis, high grade, positive margins, and T3 to 4 disease. The presence of one negative prognostic factor decreased LRR control to 37% to 63% at 10 years.

### NWHHT (Terhaard, *Int J Radiat Oncol Biol Phys* 2005)

Retrospective analysis of 498 patients treated with surgery and post-op RT or surgery alone. Post-op RT improved 10-year LC for patients with T3 to 4 tumors (84% vs. 18%), close margins (95% vs. 55%), incomplete resection (82% vs. 44%), bone invasion (86% vs. 54%), and perineural invasion (88% vs. 60%).

### UCSF cN0 Series (Chen, *Int J Radiat Oncol Biol Phys* 2007)

Retrospective analysis of 251 patients with cN0 salivary gland carcinoma treated with surgery and adjuvant RT. 131 patients (52%) received elective nodal irradiation. Elective nodal irradiation reduced the 10-year nodal failure rate from 26% to 0%. No nodal failures in patients with adenoid cystic or acinic cell histology.

### UF ACC Series (Mendenhall, *Head Neck* 2004)

Retrospective study of 101 patients with adenoid cystic carcinoma treated with RT ± surgery. The combined modality arm resulted in improved LC at 10-years (91% vs. 43%) and overall survival (OS) at 10 years (55% vs. 42%).

### UCSF ACC Series (Chen, *Int J Radiat Oncol Biol Phys* 2006)

Retrospective study of 140 patients with adenoid cystic carcinoma treated with surgery ± RT. T4 disease, perineural invasion, omission of post-op radiation, and major nerve involvement were independent predictors of LR. Among patients treated with surgery and post-op radiation, dose lower than 60 Gy, T4 disease, and major nerve involvement were predictors of LR.

# 12: LARYNX AND HYPOPHARYNX CANCERS

*Linda Chen, MD*
*Ana Kiess, MD, PhD*

## WORKUP

### All Cases

- H&P including complete head and neck exam and NPL
- Imaging—Contrast-enhanced CT or MRI of neck
- Exam under anesthesia with endoscopy as indicated
- Biopsy primary tumor and/or fine-needle aspiration (FNA) neck node
- Dental, nutrition, speech, and swallow evaluations

### Stages III to IV

- PET/CT or CT chest
- Consider PEG tube for dysphagia, weight loss, or advanced primary
- Labs: CBC, CMP, TSH

## TREATMENT RECOMMENDATIONS BY SITE AND STAGE

| | |
|---|---|
| Carcinoma in situ of glottis | Endoscopic resection (preferred) OR definitive RT |
| T1-2 N0 glottis or supraglotttis | Definitive RT OR endoscopic resection OR partial laryngectomy |
| T3-T4a N0 or N+ glottis | Definitive CRT (concurrent or induction) OR total laryngectomy (preferred for T4a) → adjuvant treatment as indicated |
| T1-2 N+ supraglottis amenable to larynx-preserving surgery | ChemoRT OR chemo → RT OR definitive RT OR partial laryngectomy → adjuvant treatment as indicated |
| T3, any N supraglottis | ChemoRT OR chemo → RT OR total laryngectomy → adjuvant treatment as indicated |

*(continued)*

| T4a, any N supraglottis | Total laryngectomy → adjuvant tx as indicated |
|---|---|
| T1N0 or select T2N0 hypopharynx amenable to larynx-preserving surgery | Definitive RT OR partial laryngopharyngectomy |
| T1 N+ or T2-3, any N hypopharynx | ChemoRT OR chemo → RT OR surgery → adjuvant tx as indicated |
| T4a, any N hypopharynx | Surgery → adjuvant tx as indicated |
| Post-op pT4, multiple positive nodes, PNI, or LVI | Adjuvant RT |
| Post-op positive margins or ECS | Adjuvant chemoRT OR re-resection for positive margins |
| T4b, any N Unresectable Unfit for surgery | Clinical trial (preferred) OR chemoRT OR chemo → RT OR definitive RT OR palliation with chemo or RT OR supportive care |
| M1 | Palliation with chemo, RT, or surgery OR supportive care |

CRT, chemoradiation with cisplatin preferred; ECS, extracapsular spread; LVI, lymphovascular invasion; PNI, perineural invasion; RT, radiation therapy.

## TECHNICAL CONSIDERATIONS

### Simulation

Simulate supine with neck extended, immobilize with thermoplastic mask. Consider bolus if there is anterior extension, superficial lymphadenopathy, or in peristomal area. Intravenous (IV) contrast if no contraindications. Fuse diagnostic or pre-op imaging.

### Dose Prescription

*Definitive RT for Early Stage Glottic Larynx*

- Cis 60.75 Gy in 2.25 Gy/fx to larynx alone
- T1N0: 63 Gy in 2.25 Gy/fx to larynx alone
- T2N0: 65.25 Gy in 2.25 Gy/fx to larynx alone

*RT for All Other Stages and Sites\**

- High-risk areas: 66 Gy in 30 fx or 70 Gy in 35 fx
- Intermediate-risk areas: 60 Gy in 30 fx or 63 Gy in 35 fx
- Low-risk areas: 54 Gy in 30 fx or 56 Gy in 35 fx

*Altered fractionation regimens such as concomitant boost or hyperfractionation are also considered

*Adjuvant RT*

- High-risk areas: 63 Gy in 30 fx or 66 Gy in 33 fx
- Intermediate-risk areas: 60 Gy in 30 fx
- Low-risk areas: 54 Gy in 30 fx

*ChemoRT*

- High-risk areas: 70 Gy in 35 fx
- Intermediate-risk areas: 63 Gy in 35 fx
- Low-risk areas: 56 Gy in 35 fx

**Target Delineation**

*Early Stage Glottic Larynx*

3DCRT with opposed laterals to larynx alone with the following borders:

- Superior: upper thyroid notch.
- Inferior: lower border of cricoid.
- Anterior: flash skin 1 cm.
- Posterior: anterior edge of vertebral body.

*Definitive RT for Other Stages and Sites*

- GTV = gross disease based on exam and imaging
- CTV high risk = GTV + margin for subclinical disease (5–10 mm)
- CTV intermediate risk (larynx) = entire larynx; levels II to IV of involved neck (+IB if II is involved; +RP if bulky nodes; +VI if subglottic extension)
- CTV intermediate risk (hypopharynx) = entire subsite of hypopharynx and nearby soft tissue/fat; entire larynx; levels IB-V + RP of involved neck
- CTV low risk = levels II to IV of uninvolved neck (+VI if subglottic extension; + RP if hypopharynx primary)
- PTV = CTV + 3- to 5-mm margin, depending on image guidance

- CTV high risk = areas of positive margins or ECE
- CTV intermediate risk = pre-op tumor bed; peristomal skin; same nodal levels as noted previously for involved neck
- CTV low risk = same nodal levels as noted previously for uninvolved neck
- PTV: CTV + 3- to 5-mm margin, depending on image guidance

## Treatment Planning
- 6-MV photons.
- For early stage glottic cancer, 3DCRT with opposed laterals is standard. Intensity-modulated radiation therapy (IMRT) for carotid sparing may be considered.
- For all other stages and sites, IMRT is preferred, with image guidance if available.

## FOLLOW UP
- PET/CT 3 months after definitive RT/CRT. If suspicion for residual disease, consider surgery. After adjuvant RT, post-treatment baseline imaging of head and neck within 6 months.
- If asymptomatic, H&P and NPL every 1 to 3 months for year 1, every 2 to 6 months for year 2, every 4 to 8 months for years 3 to 5, then annually. TSH every 6 to 12 months. Management of nutrition, dental, speech, swallow, hearing, and smoking cessation as indicated. Chest imaging as indicated for smoking history.

## SELECTED STUDIES

### VA Larynx Study (Wolf, *N Engl J Med* 1991)
Randomized trial of 332 patients with stage III to IV larynx cancer showed induction chemotherapy + definitive RT had equivalent 2-year survival rate to total laryngectomy + adjuvant RT. Induction chemotherapy + definitive RT resulted in laryngeal preservation rate of 64% at 2 years.

### EORTC 24891 (Lefebvre, *J Natl Cancer Inst* 1996)
Randomized trial of 194 patients with operable pyriform sinus or AE fold cancer showed that induction chemotherapy + definitive RT had similar control rates to surgery + adjuvant RT. Similar

rates of local failure and survival with 42% larynx preservation at 3 years.

## Japanese Glottic Cancer Trial (Yamazaki, *Int J Radiat Oncol Biol Phys* 2006)

In T1 glottic larynx cancer, a hypofractionated course with 2.25 Gy fractions (total 56.25–63 Gy) resulted in improved 5-year local control rate compared to conventional 2 Gy fractions (total 60–66 Gy). Hypofractionation associated with increased local control and no difference in 5-year cancer specific survival.

## RTOG 9111 (Forastiere, *J Clin Oncol* 2013; DOI: 10.1200/JCO.2012.43.6097)

Randomized trial of 547 patients with stage III to IV larynx cancer (excluding pts with thyroid cartilage invasion or >1 cm base of tongue invasion). Superior rates of laryngeal preservation for patients treated with concurrent CRT compared to induction chemo + RT or RT alone. Concurrent CRT reduced absolute rate of laryngectomy in follow-up. No difference in overall survival (OS) but deaths not attributed to larynx cancer or treatment were higher with concurrent CRT.

# 13: THYROID CANCER

*Ana Kiess, MD, PhD*

## WORKUP

### All Cases

- H&P including complete head and neck exam
- Imaging Neck ultrasound and fine-needle aspiration (FNA)
- Labs: TSH, T4, thyroglobulin, antithyroglobulin antibody, calcitonin
- Dental, nutrition, speech, and swallow evaluations

### Advanced Disease

- CT and/or MRI neck
- CT chest
- Nasopharyngolaryngoscopy

## TREATMENT RECOMMENDATIONS BY STAGE

### Differentiated Thyroid Cancer (DTC = Papillary, Follicular, or Hurthle Cell) or Medullary Thyroid Cancer

| | |
|---|---|
| All stages | Surgical resection of primary disease ± neck dissection |
| DTC with int-high risk per American Thyroid Association (ATA) guidelines | Consider post-op radioactive iodine (RAI) |
| Gross residual or unresectable disease (except patients <45-year old with limited RAI-avid disease) | Consider post-op external beam radiation (EBRT) |
| Patients >45 year old with microscopic residual and low likelihood of responding to RAI* | Consider post-op EBRT |
| Progressive distant metastatic disease | RAI (for DTC)<br>TSH suppression (for DTC)<br>Systemic therapy with kinase inhibitor, and/or enrollment on clinical trial<br>Consider local therapy for limited metastases |

*High likelihood of microscopic residual in patients with positive margins, extensive extracapsular nodal spread, shave excision of tumor off recurrent laryngeal nerve, trachea, or larynx, or limited esophageal resection. Low likelihood of responding to RAI in patients with recurrent disease after prior RAI, unfavorable histology, high uptake on PET, or low uptake on RAI scan. RAI is not used for medullary thyroid cancer.

## Anaplastic Thyroid Cancer

| Resectable disease, M0 | Surgical resection of primary disease ± neck dissection followed by post-op chemoRT |
| --- | --- |
| Unresectable disease, M0 | Definitive chemoRT |
| M1 | Systemic therapy OR best supportive care |

## Special Treatment Notes for Thyroid Cancer

- In the setting of microscopic residual disease, EBRT is not routine and multidisciplinary discussion is recommended.
- Cervical lymph node involvement alone should not be an indication for post-op EBRT.
- In the setting of distant metastases, overall prognosis and side effects of EBRT should be weighed against importance of locoregional control when deciding dose and volume of EBRT.

## TECHNICAL CONSIDERATIONS

### Simulation

Simulate supine with neck extended, immobilize with thermoplastic mask including shoulders. Wire scars. Consider bolus for disease near skin. Intravenous (IV) contrast only if RAI is not planned. Fuse pre-op imaging.

### Dose Prescription

- Gross disease: 70 Gy in 2 Gy/fraction
- High-risk areas: 60 to 66 Gy in 2 Gy/fraction
- Intermediate-/low-risk areas: 54 to 63 Gy in 1.6 to 1.8 Gy/fraction or 44 to 60 Gy in 2 Gy/fraction

### Target Delineation

- GTV = gross disease based on exam and imaging
- CTV high risk = areas of positive margins or shave excision
- CTV intermediate risk = areas of pre-op involvement, thyroid bed, tracheoesophageal groove, level VI nodes
- CTV low risk = uninvolved level II to V and VII nodes (in some cases, can consider not treating low-risk areas to limit toxicity)
- PTV: CTV + 3- to 5-mm margin, depending on image guidance

### Treatment Planning
- 6-MV photons
- Intensity-modulated radiation therapy (IMRT) preferred, with image guidance if available

### FOLLOW UP

Follow-up schedule, labs and imaging depend on type and stage of cancer. Discuss with endocrinologist and surgeon. Management of nutrition, dental, speech, swallow, hearing, and smoking cessation as indicated.

### SELECTED STUDIES

**2015 ATA Guidelines for Thyroid Nodules and Differentiated Thyroid Cancer (ATA Guidelines Taskforce, Haugen, *Thyroid* 2016; DOI: 10.1089/thy.2015.0020)**
Comprehensive guidelines addressing all aspects of management for patients with thyroid nodules or DTC.

**AHNS Statement on EBRT for DTC (Kiess, *Head Neck* 2016; DOI: 10.1002/hed.24357)**
Guidelines specifically addressing EBRT indications and treatment planning considerations for patients with differentiated thyroid cancer.

**EBRT for Medullary Thyroid Cancer (Terezakis, *J Natl Compr Canc Netw* 2010)**
Review article discussing EBRT for patients with medullary thyroid cancer.

# 14: OCCULT PRIMARY CANCER OF THE HEAD AND NECK

*Omar Mian, MD, PhD*
*Ana Kiess, MD, PhD*

## WORKUP

### All Cases:

- H&P including complete head and neck exam, skin exam and nasopharyngolaryngoscopy (NPL)
- Imaging—Contrast-enhanced CT or MRI of neck, PET/CT.
- Fine-needle aspiration (FNA) neck node (or core if needed)
- HPV and EBV testing on biopsy specimen. Consider thyroglobulin, calcitonin, PAX8, and/or TTF1 staining for adenocarcinoma or undifferentiated tumors.
- Dental, nutrition, speech, and swallow evaluations
- Labs: CBC, CMP, TSH
- EUA, pan-endoscopy and directed biopsies of oropharynx and any sites with clinical suspicion
- See National Comprehensive Cancer Network (NCCN) guidelines for details regarding appropriate workup

### Considerations

- If HPV+ (or HPV with upper neck nodes involved), consider palatine tonsillectomy ± lingual tonsillectomy
- If EBV+, consider nasopharynx biopsies

## TREATMENT RECOMMENDATIONS BY STAGE

| | |
|---|---|
| TX, cN1 | Neck dissection (preferred)<br>OR definitive RT<br>OR definitive ChemoRT |
| TX, cN2-3 | Neck dissection<br>OR definitive ChemoRT |
| Post-op TX, pN1<br>No ECS | Adjuvant RT<br>OR observation |
| Post-op TX, pN2-3, No ECS | Adjuvant RT (preferred)<br>OR adjuvant chemoRT |

*(continued)*

| Post-op with ECE | Adjuvant chemoRT (preferred) OR adjuvant RT |
| M1 | Platinum-based combination chemotherapy (preferred) OR clinical trial OR palliation with RT or surgery OR supportive care |

## TECHNICAL CONSIDERATIONS

### Simulation

Simulate supine with neck extended, immobilize with thermo-plastic mask. Consider mouthpiece. Wire scars. Consider bolus for disease near skin. Intravenous (IV) contrast if no contraindications. Fuse diagnostic imaging.

### Dose Prescription

- Definitive RT alone: High-risk areas: 66 Gy in 30 fx or 70 Gy in 35 fx
- Intermediate-risk areas: 60 Gy in 30 fx or 63 Gy in 35 fx
- Low-risk areas: 54 Gy in 30 fx or 56 Gy in 35 fx
- Adjuvant RT: High-risk areas: 63 Gy in 30 fx, or 66 Gy in 33 fx
- Intermediate-risk areas: 60 Gy in 30 fx
- Low-risk areas: 54 Gy in 30 fx
- ChemoRT: High-risk areas: 70 Gy in 35 fx
- Intermediate-risk areas: 63 Gy in 35 fx
- Low-risk areas: 56 Gy in 35 fx

### Target Delineation

- GTV = gross disease based on exam and imaging
- CTV high risk = GTV + margin for subclinical disease (5–10 mm)
- CTV intermediate risk:
  - Central: CTV for central structures is determined by tumor size, nodal stations and HPV/EBV. Historically included entire pharynx and larynx.
  - Neck: Bilateral IB-V and RP if bilateral neck involvement. Ipsilateral IB-V and RP if only ipsilateral neck involvement.

- CTV low risk = uninvolved contralateral II to IV nodes (cannot omit)
- PTV = CTV + 3- to 5-mm margin, depending on image guidance

**Treatment Planning**
- 6-MV photons
- Intensity-modulated radiation therapy (IMRT) preferred, with image guidance if available.

**FOLLOW UP**

PET/CT 3 months after definitive RT/CRT. If suspicion for residual neck disease, consider neck dissection. After adjuvant RT, posttreatment baseline imaging of head and neck within 6 months.

If asymptomatic, H&P and NPL every 1 to 3 months for year 1, every 2 to 6 months for year 2, every 4 to 8 months for years 3 to 5, then annually. TSH every 6 to 12 months. Low threshold for biopsy if suspect emergence of primary. Management of nutrition, dental, speech, swallow, hearing, and smoking cessation as indicated. Chest imaging as indicated for smoking history.

**SELECTED STUDIES**

**Occult Primary Site Detection (Cianchetti, *Layngoscope* 2009; DOI: 10.1002/lary.20638)**
236 patients with occult primary underwent CT, MRI, panendoscopy with directed biopsies, PET, and/or tonsillectomies. Occult primary was detected in 53% with the majority of these found in the tonsil (45%) and base of tongue (44%).

**Bilateral Tonsillectomy (Koch, *Otolaryngol Head Neck Surg* 2001)**
Oncologic rationale for bilateral tonsillectomy in head and neck squamous cell carcinoma of unknown primary. Rate of contralateral tonsil primary approaches 10%.

**EORTC 22931 and RTOG 9501 (Bernier, *Head Neck* 2005)**
CRT improved disease-free survival and local/regional control in patients with ECE or positive margins, but provided only trend for

improvements in stage III to IV, PNI, LVSI, and/or enlarged level IV to V nodes. Patients with $\geq 2$ involved nodes without ECE as their only risk factor did not benefit from chemo.

## Cancer of Unknown Primary Treated With IMRT
(Shoushtari, *Int J Radiat Oncol Biol Phys* 2011; DOI: 10.1016/j.ijrobp.2011.01.014)

Definitive IMRT and neck dissection results in excellent nodal control and overall and disease-free survival with acceptable toxicity for patients with T0N1 or T0N2a disease without ECS.

# 15: NONSMALL CELL LUNG CANCER

*Daniel D. Chamberlain, MD*

## WORKUP

### All Cases

- H&P (include weight loss and performance status)
- Smoking cessation assistance
- Pulmonary function tests
- PET/CT
- Bronchoscopy
- Consider pathologic evaluation of mediastinal nodes
- Pathologic confirmation

### If Stage >IA

- Pathologic evaluation of mediastinal nodes
- MRI brain

### If Superior Sulcus Tumor Abutting Spine or Subclavian Vessels

- MRI spine and thoracic inlet

### If Stage IV

- Genomic testing (e.g., EGFR, ALK, ROS1) particularly for adenocarcinoma, but may include squamous cell carcinoma in patients with minimal tobacco history

## TREATMENT RECOMMENDATIONS BY STAGE

| IA | Surgery (lobectomy + node dissection preferred) |
|---|---|
| IA inoperable | SBRT is an alternative to limited (sublobar)surgery |
| IB | Surgery → ±chemo (in select cases) |
| IB inoperable | SBRT → ±chemo (in select cases) |
| IIA | Surgery → chemo |
| IIA inoperable | ChemoRT |
| IIB | Surgery → chemo |
| IIB inoperable | ChemoRT |
| IIIA | Neoadjuvant chemoRT → Surgery → Chemo<br>OR chemo → Surgery → RT<br>OR definitive ChemoRT |

*(continued)*

*(continued)*

| IIIA Resectable T3-4, N0-1 | Surgery → Chemo |
| IIIA Unable to tolerate concurrent treatment | Sequential radiation and chemotherapy |
| IIIB | ChemoRT |
| IIIB Tumor too large for RT | Chemo → reevaluate for ChemoRT |
| IIIB Unable to tolerate concurrent tx | Sequential therapy or systemic therapy alone |
| IV | Systemic therapy |
| IV (M1a) effusion | Systemic therapy. In cases where the fluid is repeatedly path negative may consider definitive therapy |
| IV (M1b) single brain or adrenal met | Consider definitive treatment to the met and thoracic disease |
| IV (M1a) Solitary contralateral lung | Treat as separate primaries |
| Multiple lung cancers (>2) | Local therapy if symptomatic, at risk of becoming symptomatic, or solitary metachronous lesion. Otherwise chemo. |
| Superior sulcus T3N0-N1 resectable | Neoadjuvant chemoRT → Surgery → Chemo |
| Superior sulcus T4 N0-N1 borderline resectable | ChemoRT → rapid evaluation → (surgery if resectable → Chemo) versus finish definitive chemoRT |
| Superior sulcus unresectable | Definitive chemoRT |
| Post-op pN0-N1 | Chemotherapy as appropriate per stage |
| Post-op pN2 | Chemotherapy → Post-op radiation |
| Post-op Margin + | ChemoRT |

## TECHNICAL CONSIDERATIONS

### Simulation
- Supine, arms up, immobilization
- Simulate and treat with respiratory motion assessment and management strategy (e.g., 4DCT and ITV or gating)

## Dose Prescription
- SBRT: BED10 >100 54 Gy in 3 fx, 50 Gy in 4 fx, 50 Gy in 5 fx
- Definitive chemo-RT: 60 to 66 Gy in 30 to 33 fx
- Pre-op chemo-RT: 45 to 50 Gy in 25 fx
- Post-op RT: 50 to 54 Gy in 25 to 30 fx at 1.8 to 2 Gy/fx

## Target Delineation
- Contour parenchymal lesions on lung window, lymphnodes on a soft tissue window.
- GTV based on imaging and biopsies
- ITV = GTV contoured in all phases of respiration to obtain iGTV, then + 8 mm for clinical target volume (CTV) expansion *OR* GTV+ 8 mm to obtain CTV and then contour CTV in all phases of respiration)
- PTV = ITV + 0.3 to 0.5 cm depending on localization method and reproducibility
- Limiting treatment to tumor and involved nodal stations is preferred over radiation of elective (uninvolved) nodal areas.
- In post-op cases include the hilar stump in the CTV.
- For SBRT PTV= iGTV (GTV on all phases of respiration) + 5 mm (no CTV expansion)
- Daily CBCT

## Planning
- 6- to 10-MV photons
- Heterogeneity corrections used
- Intensity-modulated radiation therapy (IMRT) may improve patient reported quality of life.

## FOLLOW UP

If asymptomatic: CT chest and H&P Q6 months × 2 years then annually.

## SELECTED STUDIES

### RTOG 0236 (Timmerman, *JAMA* 2010; DOI: 10.1001/jama.2010.261)
59 patients with NSCLC T1-2N0 tumor <5 cm treated with 54 Gy in 3 fx. Three-year LC 97.6%, 3-year overall survival (OS) =55.8%

### Intergroup 0139 (Albain, *Lancet* 2009; DOI: 10.1016/S0140-6736(09)60737-6)
369 patients with T1-3N2 NSCLC randomized to concurrent chemoRT 45 Gy then surgery (if no progression) then chemo

× 2 cycles versus concurrent chemoRT 61 Gy. No difference in OS. Progression-free survival (PFS) improved in surgery arm. In exploratory analysis, OS improved in patients randomized to surgery if they underwent lobectomy, but not pneumonectomy.

### SEER PORT study (Lally, *J Clin Oncol* 2006)

SEER review of 7,400 stage II to III NSCLC patients s/p lobectomy or pneumonectomy. Increased use of PORT correlated to T3 to T4, tumor size, node stage, number of involved nodes, and ratio involved nodes to sampled nodes. Subset analysis for patients with N2 disease ([HR] 0.855; 95% CI, [0.762, 0.959]; $P = .0077$), PORT was associated with a significant increase in survival. Survival worse for N0 patients treated with PORT

### RTOG 0617 (Bradley, *Lancet Oncology* 2015; DOI: 10.1016/S1470-2045(14)71207-0)

Randomized 464 stage III patients to concurrent chemoRT to either 60 Gy of 74 Gy. MS (28.7 vs. 19.5 months) and OS at 18 months (66.9% vs. 53.9%) favored 60 Gy. Fewer local regional failures (35.3% vs. 44%) in the 60 Gy arm. Patient reported QOL better in patients treated with IMRT in both arms.

### LAMP (Belani, *J Clin Oncol* 2005)

Patients with stage III NSCLC randomized to: induction chemo × 2 cycles then RT 63 Gy, versus induction chemo × 2 cycles then concurrent chemoRT 63 Gy, versus concurrent chemoRT 63 Gy then paclitaxel/carboplatin × 2 cycles consolidation. Median OS (13.0, 12.7, and 16.3 months) favored upfront concurrent chemoRT.

### HOG (Hanna, *J Clin Oncol* 2008; DOI: 10.1200/JCO.2008.17.7840)

Stage III NSCLC patients treated with concurrent chemoRT 59.4 Gy then if no progression randomized to consolidation docetaxel versus observation. Stopped early after analysis of 203 patients. Increased toxicity but no survival benefit from consolidation chemo.

### Intergroup 0160 (Rusch, *J Clin Oncol* 2007)

110 patients with T3 to T4, N0-1 Superior sulcus NSCLC treated with concurrent chemoRT 45 Gy then (if no progression) surgery, then chemo × 2 cycles. Eighty percent underwent surgery and 76% had R0 resection. Unresectable patients had completion chemoRT to 63 Gy total. 5-year OS.

# 16: SMALL CELL LUNG CANCER

*Brandon R. Mancini, MD*
*Roy H. Decker, MD, PhD*

## WORKUP

### All Cases

- H&P (include weight loss and performance status)
- Smoking cessation assistance
- MRI brain
- PET/CT
- CBC with differential and platelets
- Electrolytes, LFTs, Ca, LDH
- BUN, creatinine
- Pathologic confirmation

### Considerations

- Pathologic evaluation of mediastinal nodes
- Thoracentesis with cytopathology for pleural effusions
- Bone marrow biopsy (for metastatic patients with elevated LDH)
- Bone scan if PET available
- PFTs

## TREATMENT RECOMMENDATIONS BY STAGE*

| IA | Surgery (lobectomy + node dissection preferred) for peripheral nodules → platinum-based chemotherapy → Prophylactic Cranial Irradiation (PCI) OR chemoRT → PCI |
|---|---|
| IA inoperable | ChemoRT → PCI |
| IB | Surgery (lobectomy + node dissection preferred) for peripheral nodules → platinum-based chemotherapy → PCI ChemoRT → PCI |
| IA inoperable | ChemoRT → PCI |
| IIA | ChemoRT → PCI |
| IIB | ChemoRT → PCI |
| IIIA | ChemoRT → PCI |

*(continued)*

| IIIA unable to tolerate concurrent | Sequential chemotherapy and radiation therapy ➜ PCI |
|---|---|
| IIIB | ChemoRT ➜ PCI |
| IIIB tumor too large for RT | Chemo ➜ re-evaluate for ChemoRT ➜ PCI<br>Sequential chemotherapy and radiation therapy ➜ PCI |
| IIIB unable to tolerate concurrent | Sequential chemotherapy and radiation therapy ➜ PCI |
| IV | Chemo ➜ PCI ± thoracic RT if good response to chemo |

*1. Limited-stage: AJCC (7th Edition) Stage I to III (T any, N any, M0) that can be treated with definitive radiation doses safely. Excludes T3 to 4 due to multiple lung nodules or tumor/nodal volume too large to be encompassed in a safe and tolerable radiation plan.

2. Extensive-stage: AJCC (7th Edition) Stage IV (T any, N any, M1a/b), or T3 to 4 due to multiple lung nodules too extensive or have tumor/nodal volume too large to be encompassed in a safe and tolerable radiation plan.

## TECHNICAL CONSIDERATIONS

### Simulation
Simulate and treat with respiratory motion assessment and management strategy (e.g., 4DCT and ITV or gating). PET/CT simulation can be considered when available

### Dose Prescription
- Definitive ChemoRT: 45 Gy in 30 fx at 1.5 Gy/fx BID or 60 to 70 Gy in 30 to 35 fx at 2 Gy/fx daily
- PCI: 25 Gy in 10 fractions at 2.5 Gy/fx
- Thoracic RT in extensive stage: 30 Gy in 10 fx.

### Target Delineation
- Contour parenchymal lesions on lung windows, nodes on a soft tissue window.
- GTV = gross disease based on imaging and biopsies
- ITV = GTV contoured on all phases of respiration to obtain iGTV, then + 8 mm for clinical target volume (CTV) expansion *OR* GTV+ 8 mm to obtain CTV and then contour CTV in all phases of respiration

- PTV = ITV + set up error 3 to 5 mm
- Limiting treatment to tumor and involved nodal stations is preferred over radiation of elective (uninvolved) nodal areas.
- If using free-breathing, non-ITV volume, PTV is CTV + 1.5 (superior–inferior direction) and 1.0 cm (radially).
- Daily kV or CBCT imaging.

### Treatment Planning
- 6- to 10-MV photons
- Heterogeneity corrections used
- Intensity-modulated radiation therapy (IMRT) may improve patient reported quality of life, reduce dose to organs at risk, or allow higher prescription dose to selected patients

### FOLLOW UP

If asymptomatic: H&P, CT Chest, and labs at each visit. Visits q2 to 3 months for year 1, q3 to 4 months for years 2 to 3, q4 to 6 months for years 4 to 5, then annually thereafter.

PET scan should be considered if CT findings suggest recurrence or metastases.

### SELECTED STUDIES

#### INT-0096 (Turrisi, *N Engl J Med* 1999)
Randomized 381 patients with limited-stage SCLC treated with platinum and etoposide (EP) × 4 cycles and RT at first cycle to 1.5 Gy BID × 3 weeks versus 1.8 Gy daily × 5 weeks (both to 45 Gy), followed by PCI to 25 Gy. Better 5-year overall survival (OS) (26% vs. 16%) and LC (64% vs. 48%) in BID arm. Increased grade 3 esophagitis (27% vs. 11%) with BID regimen.

#### CALGB 39808 (Bogart, *Int J Radiat Oncol Biol Phys* 2004)
57 patients treated with thoracic radiation therapy after receiving two cycles of induction chemotherapy with paclitaxel/topotecan followed by three cycles of carboplatin/etoposide. Thoracic RT 70 Gy in 35 fx over 7 weeks initiated with first cycle of carboplatin/etoposide. 2-year OS 48% and FFS 31%. Grade 3+ dysphagia 21%.

#### Role of Radiation Therapy in the Combined-Modality Treatment of Patients With Extensive Disease Small-Cell Lung Cancer: A Randomized Study (Jeremic, *J Clin Oncol* 1999)
210 patients treated with three cycles of EP. Patients with a local and distant CR a local PR and a distant CR were randomized to

thoracic RT 54 Gy in 36 fx over 18 tx days with carboplatin/etoposide followed by two cycles of EP versus an additional four cycles of EP alone. Better 5-year OS (9.1% vs. 3.7%) in thoracic RT group.

### Systematic Review Evaluating the Timing of Thoracic Radiation Therapy in Combined Modality Therapy for Limited-Stage Small-Cell Lung Cancer (Fried, *J Clin Oncol* 2004)

Meta-analysis of seven randomized trials of patients with limited-stage SCLC evaluating the timing of thoracic RT. Patients were separated based on early (<9 weeks after initiation of chemotherapy) versus late (≥9 weeks) commencement of thoracic RT. There was a 5.2% absolute 2-year OS with early RT. Benefit more pronounced with cisplatin-based chemotherapy.

### Use of Thoracic Radiotherapy for Extensive Stage Small-Cell Lung Cancer: A Phase 3 Randomized Controlled Trial (Slotman, *Lancet* 2015; DOI: 10.1016/S0140-6736(14)61085-0)

Randomized 495 patients with extensive-stage SCLC who responded to chemotherapy to thoracic RT (30 Gy in 10 fx) versus no thoracic RT. All patients received PCI. Better 2-year OS (13% vs. 3%) on secondary analysis. No significant difference in 1-year OS between groups (33% vs. 28%). Better 6-month progression-free survival (PFS) in thoracic RT group (24% vs. 7%).

### Prophylactic Cranial Irradiation for Patients With Small-Cell Lung Cancer in Complete Remission (Auperin, *N Engl J Med* 1999)

Meta-analysis of seven randomized controlled trials comparing PCI versus no PCI after CR after induction chemotherapy ± RT and no evidence of brain metastases prior to randomization. Better 3-year OS (20.7% vs. 15.3%) and decreased 3-year incidence of brain metastases (33% vs. 59%) with PCI.

### EORTC 08993 (Slotman, *N Engl J Med* 2007)

286 patients with extensive-stage SCLC treated with chemotherapy randomized to PCI versus no PCI after any response to chemotherapy and primary end point was time to symptomatic brain metastases. Most patients received 20 Gy in 5 fx. PCI decreased 1-year incidence of symptomatic brain metastases (15% vs. 40%). Better 1-year OS (27% vs. 13%) with PCI.

# 17: MESOTHELIOMA

*Brandon R. Mancini, MD*
*Roy H. Decker, MD, PhD*

## WORKUP

### All Cases
- H&P
- Thoracentesis for cytologic assessment
- Pleural biopsy for pathologic confirmation
- PFTs
- Imaging—CT chest/abdomen with contrast, PET/CT
- Labs—CBC, CMP, LDH

### Considerations
- Soluble mesothelin-related peptide
- Osteopontin level
- Chest MRI
- Mediastinoscopy/EBUS fine-needle aspiration (FNA) for pathologic evaluation of mediastinal nodes
- VATS and/or laparoscopy if concern of contralateral or peritoneal disease
- Talc pleurodesis or a pleural catheter if effusion
- Cardiac stress test (surgical evaluation)

## TREATMENT RECOMMENDATIONS BY STAGE

| I to III<br>Epithelial or mixed | *Surgery → Chemo ± RT<br>OR chemo → *Surgery ± RT<br>OR chemotherapy |
|---|---|
| I to III, Sarcomatoid<br>IV | Chemotherapy |
| Medically inoperable | Observation if poor PS<br>OR chemotherapy |
| Unresectable | Chemo → reevaluate *surgery<br>OR chemo |

*Surgery includes either extrapleural pneumonectomy (EPP) or pleurectomy/decortication

## TECHNICAL CONSIDERATIONS

### Simulation

- Simulate and treat with respiratory motion assessment and management strategy (e.g., 4DCT and ITV or gating)
- Wire all instrumentation scars

### Dose Prescription

- Hemi-thoracic RT after EPP
  - Negative margins: 50 to 54 Gy in 25 to 30 fx
  - Micro–macroscopic + margins: 54 to 60 Gy in 30 fx
- Palliative for chest wall pain: 20 to 40 Gy in >4 Gy/fx or 30 Gy in 10 fx
- Doses of ≥60 Gy for macroscopic tumors (if tolerable)
- Prophylactic radiation to surgical sites: 21 Gy in 7 fx

### Target Delineation

- GTV based on imaging, and biopsies
- CTV = in addition to GTV with appropriate expansion it must include entire pleural surface (for partial resection cases) from thoracic inlet to diaphragmatic insertion, ipsilateral mediatinal/hilar lymph nodes, surgical clips, as well as all incision and surgical drain sites
- PTV = 1 to 1.5 cm expansion on CTV
- Ensure coverage of anteromedial pleura, which can cross midline

### Treatment Planning

- 3DCRT or intensity-modulated radiation therapy (IMRT)
- 6- to 10-MV mixed energy photons, electrons
- IMRT with parenchymal sparing may be considered after pleurectomy

## FOLLOW UP

If asymptomatic: Frequent follow-up visits with CT chest and H&P indefinitely.

## SELECTED STUDIES

### EORTC 08031 (Van Schil, *Eur Respir J*, 2010; DOI: 10.1183/09031936.00039510)

Phase II trial of 58 patients investigating the feasibility of tri-modality therapy consisting of induction chemotherapy (cisplatin/pemetrexed) → extrapleural pneumonectomy → post-op radiotherapy (54 Gy in 30 fractions) in patients with malignant pleural mesothelioma. 37 patients completed RT. Local recurrence 16% in patients completing all trimodality therapy. Median overall survival (OS) is 18.4 months.

### MSKCC Phase II Trial (Rusch, *J Thorac Cardiovasc Surg* 2001)

Phase II trial of 88 patients who underwent hemithorax RT (54 Gy) after EPP. Seventy percent of patients had EPP. Improved local control and survival compared to historical controls. RT decreased rate of LR. 2-year OS 33%. MS 34 months for stages I to II and 10 months for stages III to IV.

### Harvard Retrospective Review (Sugarbaker, *J Thorac Cardiovasc Surg* 1999)

Retrospective review of 183 patients treated with EPP + adjuvant chemotherapy (Cytoxan/Adriamycin/cisplatin or carboplatin/Taxol) + RT (30 Gy in 20 fx at 1.5 Gy/fx to hemithorax with boost to 50.4 Gy w/concurrent Taxol) ➔ adjuvant chemotherapy. MS 19 months. 5-year OS 15%. Factors for better outcomes included epithelial histology, negative resection margins, and negative extrapleural lymph nodes. If all three positive prognostic factors, 5-year OS 46%.

### MDACC IMRT Experience (Rice, *Int J Radiat Oncol Biol Phys* 2007)

Retrospective review of 63 patients who underwent IMRT after EPP (doses 45–50 Gy). Contralateral lung V20 was predictor of pulmonary-related death. If >7%, 42 × risk of death. 9% of patients with fatal pulmonary death related to V20.

### MSKCC 3D Experience (Yajnik, *Int J Radiat Oncol Biol Phys* 2003)

Retrospective review of 35 patients who underwent hemithoracic 3DCRT after EPP to a doses from 45 to 54 Gy. A combined AP/PA photon/electron plan is described.

### Pemetrexed Trial (Vogelzang, *J Clin Oncol* 2003)

Phase III study of 456 patients with MPM randomized to pemetrexed in combination with cisplatin versus cisplatin alone. Improved median OS in pemetrexed arm (12.1 vs. 9.3 months). Response rate of 41.3% in pemetrexed arm versus 16.7% in cisplatin alone arm. Folic acid and vitamin B12 supplementation added with subsequent reduced treatment toxicity.

# 18: THYMOMA

*Brandon R. Mancini, MD*
*Roy H. Decker, MD, PhD*

## WORKUP

### All Cases

- H&P (include B symptoms [fever >38°C, night sweats, >10% weight loss in preceding 6 months] and symptoms of myasthenia gravis [easy fatigability, ptosis, diplopia])
- Imaging—CXR, CT chest with contrast
- Labs—CBC, platelets, LDH, ESR, AFP/HCG
- Pathologic confirmation

### Considerations

- Tensilon test
- PET/CT
- MRI chest
- Pulmonary function tests

## TREATMENT RECOMMENDATIONS BY MODIFIED MASAOKA STAGE

| I | Surgery |
|---|---|
| IIA | Surgery |
| IIB | Surgery |
| IIIA | Surgery ±RT<br>OR Chemo → Surgery<br>OR Chemo → RT ± chemo |
| IIIB | Surgery → ±RT<br>OR Chemo → Surgery<br>OR Chemo → RT ± chemo |
| IVA (limited pleural disease) | Surgery → ±RT or Chemo<br>OR Surgery → Chemo<br>OR Chemo → Surgery<br>OR Chemo → RT ± chemo |
| IVA (disseminated pleural disease) or IVB | Chemo alone |

(continued)

| Post-op without microscopic residual tumor (R0) | No further therapy for stage I or II<br>Consider RT for stage III,IV<br>RT + chemotherapy for thymic carcinoma |
|---|---|
| Post-op w/ microscopic residual tumor (R1) | RT<br>OR RT ± chemo if thymic carcinoma |
| Post-op w/ macroscopic residual tumor (R2) | RT ± chemo<br>OR RT + chemo if thymic carcinoma |

## TECHNICAL CONSIDERATIONS

### Simulation

Simulate and treat with respiratory motion management and assessment strategy (e.g., 4DCT and ITV or gating) if indicated.

### Dose Prescription

- Definitive RT (unresectable disease): 60 to 70 Gy in 1.8 to 2 Gy/fx
- Adjuvant RT for clear/close margins: 45 to 50 Gy in 1.8 to 2 Gy/fx
- Microscopically positive margins: 54 Gy in 1.8 to 2 Gy/fx
- Gross residual disease: ≥60 Gy in 1.8 to 2 Gy/fx

### Target Delineation

- Contour on a soft tissue window
- GTV based on imaging and biopsies
- CTV = encompass the entire thymus (for partial resection cases), surgical clips, and any potential sites with residual disease; reviewed with thoracic surgeon
- PTV = consider daily target motion and setup error; exact margin based on individual patient's motion, simulation technique, and reproducibility of setup

### Treatment Planning

- 3D conformal or intensity-modulated radiation therapy (IMRT) should be utilized
- IMRT may improve patient reported quality of life
- 6- to 10-MV photons

## FOLLOW UP

If asymptomatic: CT and H&P every 6 months × 2 years, then annually × 5 years for thymic carcinoma and 10 years for thymoma.

## SELECTED STUDIES

### Post-Op Radiotherapy for Stage I Thymoma (Zhang, *Chin Med J* 1999)

29 patients with stage I thymoma, age <65 years, randomized to surgery alone versus surgery + adjuvant RT. There was no recurrence or metastases in either group. 10-year overall survival (OS) was 92% versus 88% in surgery versus surgery + adjuvant RT cohorts, respectively. Authors conclude that adjuvant RT not necessary for stage I thymoma.

### SEER (Forquer, *Int J Radiat Oncol Biol Phys* 2010; DOI: 10.1016/j.ijrobp.2009.02.016)

SEER review of 901 patients with surgically resected thymoma or thymic carcinoma. Patients analyzed according to Masaoka stage. Post-op RT was received by 65% of patients. Masaoka Stage I (localized)—RT may adversely impact 5-year cause-specific survival (PORT 91% vs. No PORT 98%). Masaoka Stage II to III (regional)—5-year CSS 91% versus 86% (NS). 5-year OS 76% versus 66%. Overall post-op RT with no benefit in Masaoka Stage I, possible OS benefit in stage II to III.

### Adjuvant Radiotherapy for Thymic Epithelial Tumor: Treatment Results and Prognostic Factors (Kundel, *Am J Clin Oncol* 2007)

Retrospective study of 47 thymic tumors treated with adjuvant RT. RT dose 26 to 60 Gy. Median follow-up 10.6 years. 5-year OS 73% (77% thymoma vs. 33% thymic carcinoma). Stage II 5-year OS: RT dose ≤45 Gy 59% versus >45 Gy 100%; DFS 37% versus 100%. Lower stage (II vs. III/IV), surgery (resection vs. biopsy), higher RT dose (≤45 vs. >45 Gy) predicted OS. Thymic carcinoma histology no impact on OS, only DFS. Authors conclude post-op RT should be >45 Gy.

### Concurrent Chemoradiotherapy for Unresectable Thymic Carcinoma (Chen, *Chang Gung Med J* 2004)

Retrospective review of 16 patients treated with concurrent chemoradiotherapy for unresectable thymic carcinoma. Chemotherapy consisted of cisplatin + 5-FU or doxorubicin, cisplatin, vincristine and cyclophosphamide. RT given concurrently from 34.2 to 70 Gy. 25.0% with complete response, 25% with partial response, 37.5% with stable disease, and 12.5% with progression. Overall response rate 50%. Median OS 82 months.

# 19: EARLY STAGE BREAST CANCER

*Sanjay Aneja, MD*
*Adam Kole, MD, PhD*
*Meena Moran, MD*

## WORKUP

- H&P (include gynecologic, family history)
- Diagnostic bilateral mammogram, breast ultrasound, biopsy of primary tumor and any clinically suspicious axillary nodes
- Breast MRI (optional)
- Path: Primary tumor size, histology, grade, margins, multifocality, estrogen receptor/progesterone receptor (ER/PR), Her2-neu, LVSI, nodes removed, nodes involved, ECE
- Consider labs (CBC, LFTs, alk phos, etc.) or metastatic work-up (chest CT, bone scan, PET/CT) as directed by signs/symptoms, or for clinical stage IIIA (T3, N1) or greater
- Genetic counseling if high risk (triple negative breast cancer and <60 years old, early-age onset breast cancer, known mutation in family, multiple primary cancers, criteria for personal and family history)
- Fertility counseling if premenopausal

## TREATMENT RECOMMENDATIONS BY STAGE

| 0 (Ductal carcinoma in situ [DCIS]) | Breast-conserving surgery → RT → Endocrine therapy for ER/PR+<br>Consider mastectomy + sentinel lymph node biopsy (SLNB) for multicentric disease, persistently + margins, large volume DCIS relative to breast size → Endocrine therapy for ER/PR+ |
|---|---|
| Stage I to II (T1-2N0) | BCS and SLNB → Chemotherapy if high-risk disease[a] → RT → Endocrine therapy if ER/PR+ OR Mastectomy and surgical evaluation of axillary nodes → Chemotherapy if high-risk disease[a] → Endocrine therapy for ER/PR+<br>Consider neoadjuvant chemotherapy for downsizing for larger tumors |

[a]Triple negative breast cancer/Her2+/Oncotype high risk.

## Margin Status Following Breast Conservation
- **DCIS:** ≥2 mm
- **Invasive Disease:** No tumor on ink

## National Comprehensive Cancer Network Contraindications to Breast Conservation With RT
- **Absolute:** Pregnancy, diffuse microcalcifications suspicious for malignancy, inability to achieve good cosmesis (large tumor relative to breast size)
- **Relative:** Prior ipsilateral RT, scleroderma/lupus, T3 tumors, genetic predisposition to breast cancer

## Oncotype Dx Score: Initial Validation of ER(+) Node (–) Tumors
Low risk (0–17) ➜ No benefit
   Intermediate risk (18–30) ➜ consider chemotherapy
   High risk (>30) ➜ benefit to chemotherapy

## Omission of RT Following Breast-Conserving Surgery
- **DCIS:** Consider only in select patients with advanced age/comorbidities, or small, low-grade lesions with widely negative margins (Eastern Cooperative Oncology Group [ECOG] 5194; DOI: 10.1200/JCO.2015.60.8588)
- **Invasive Disease:** Consider in ER+ elderly patients, ages >65 to 70, with primary tumors <2 to 3 cm, willing to take adjuvant hormonal therapy (Cancer and Leukemia Group B [CALGB] 9343, PRIME II; DOI: 10.1016/j.clon.2004.07.008)

## TECHNICAL CONSIDERATIONS

### Simulation
Standard: supine position (breast board or alpha cradle), arms up, clinical breast borders and surgical scar wired.
   Technical considerations for decreasing lung and/or heart dose:

- Heart block (ensure breast tissue at risk is not blocked)
- Prone positioning (breast tangents only)
- Deep inspiration breath-hold

### Dose Prescription
*Conventionally Fractionated Whole Breast Radiation Therapy*
- Breast: 50 to 50.4 Gy in 25 to 28 fx Boost: 10 to 16 Gy in 5 to 8 fx

*Hypofractionated Fractionated Whole Breast Radiation Therapy*
- American Society for Radiation Oncology (ASTRO) Recommendations (2011): T1-2N0, age >50 years, post lumpectomy, no chemo, dose inhomogeneity 93% to 107%, without regional nodal RT fields
- Breast: 40.05 Gy in 15 fx or 42.7 Gy in 16 fx Boost: 10 Gy in 4 to 5 fx

*Accelerated Partial Breast Irradiation*
- ASTRO Guidelines (2011): Age >60, pT1N0 (must have nodal evaluation), only invasive ductal carcinoma (IDC), margins ≥2 mm, ER(+), No LVI, multifocality or extensive intraductal component (EIC). External beam radiation therapy (EBRT) dose: 38.5 Gy in 10 fx over 5 days (twice a day [BID]) to cavity + 2.5 cm. Brachytherapy dose: 34 Gy in 10 fx over 5 days (BID) to cavity + 1 cm.

**Target Delineation**
Contour organs at risk, breast volumes, nodal targets (Radiation Therapy Oncology Group [RTOG] Breast Contouring Atlas). Based on clinical and radiographic volumes:

- CTV = as defined by RTOG Atlas and/or clinical volumes at risk
- PTV = Breast/Chest wall CTV + 7–mm expansion (excludes heart and does not cross midline).
- PTV Eval = Subtracts PTV extending into lung (or chest wall for breast-conserving cases) and 3 to 5 mm off of skin anteriorly (buildup region)

**Treatment Planning**
- **Beam Energies:** 6-MV to 18-MV photons (often used in combination)
- **Beam Arrangements:** Tangential fields with forward planned or inverse planned segments to achieve **treatment goals/constraints**:
    - **Cardiac:** $V_{\geq 20\,Gy} \leq 5\%$; $V_{\geq 10\,Gy} \leq 30\%$; Heart Dose$_{Mean}$: <400 cGy
    - **Lung:** $V_{20Gy} < 15\%$, $V_{10\,Gy} < 35\%$
    - **Whole breast PTV Eval:** $V_{\geq 95\%} \geq 95\%$; Max dose <115%, $V_{108\%} \leq 50\%$.

## FOLLOW UP

If asymptomatic: History and physical exam every 3 to 12 months as appropriate. Diagnostic mammogram annually. No routine imaging of reconstructed breast indicated.

## SELECTED STUDIES (DCIS)

### Early Breast Cancer Trialists' Collaborative Group Meta-analysis of RT Following BCS for DCIS (Early Breast Cancer Trialists' Collaborative Group (EBCTCG), *J Natl Cancer Inst Monogr* 2010; DOI: 10.1093/jncimonographs/lgq039)

Meta-analysis of randomized DCIS clinical trials. BCS+RT associated with reduced ipsilateral breast tumor recurrence (IBTR) at 5 years (7.6% vs. 18.1%) and 10 years (12.9% vs. 28.1%). The benefit was seen regardless of age, grade, size, and tamoxifen use. No overall survival benefit with RT.

### American College of Surgeons Oncology Group Z0011 Trial (Giuliano et al., *JAMA* 2011; DOI: 10.1001/jama.2011.90)

Phase III noninferiority trial: cT1-2N0, pN1 with 1 to 2 + sentinel lymph node (SLN) randomized to ± axillary lymph node dissection (ALND) before whole breast radiation therapy. No differences in 5 years axillary relapse rates, OS, or DFS with or without ALND. Of note, protocol specified breast radiation alone, but review of a subset of port films revealed significant variations in both arms receiving directed nodal RT (high tangent or third field) (Jagsi et. al., *J Clin Oncol* 2014; DOI: 10.1200/JCO.2014.56.5838).

### RTOG 98-04: Observation RT for DCIS (McCormick, *J Clin Oncol* 2015; DOI: 10.1200/JCO.2014.57.9029)

Prospective randomized trial of BCS with or without radiation for low-risk DCIS, defined as low-/intermediate-grade DCIS <2.5 cm in size with margins ≥ 3 mm. Despite closure of trial due to poor accrual, the 7-year follow-up of the 636 patients enrolled demonstrated a statistically significant benefit of RT in decreasing IBTR (0.9% RT vs. 6.7% no RT ($P < .001$).

## SELECTED STUDIES (EARLY–STAGE INVASIVE)

### EBCTCG Meta-Analysis of Adjuvant RT Following BCS (EBCTCG, *Lancet* 2011; DOI: 10.1016/S0140-6736(11)61629-2)

Meta-analysis of 17 studies and 10,801 patients. For pN0, RT following lumpectomy associated with a 15% absolute risk reduction of 10-year local or distant recurrence (16% vs. 31.0%) and with 3% cancer-specific survival benefit at 15 years (17% vs. 21%).

### Margin Status Following BCS (Moran et al., *J Clin Oncol* 2014; DOI: 10.1200/JCO.2013.53.3935)

Meta-analysis of IBTR risk and margin widths from 33 studies and 28,162 invasive breast cancer patients after BCS + RT. Positive margin following BCS (tumor on ink) associated with twofold increase in risk of IBTR (odds ratio [OR] 2.44) regardless of favorable biology, receipt of systemic therapy, or radiation therapy boost. Consensus panel concluded based on meta-analysis and aggregate data on current IBTR that negative margins should be defined as no ink on tumor.

### ASTRO Consensus Guidelines for Hypofractionated RT (Smith et al., *Int J Radiat Oncol Biol Phys* 2011; DOI: 10.1016/j.ijrobp.2010.04.042)

Systematic review of literature and consensus recommendations of hypofractionation regimens in early-stage breast cancer. Recommendation: hypofractionation suitable in women aged >50, stage pT1-2N0, who did not receive chemotherapy, and could receive radiation with 7% dose homogeneity.

### Cancer and Leukemia Group B (CALGB) 9343: BCS+ Tamoxifen for ER+ patients Age >70 (Hughes et al., *J Clin Oncol* 2013; DOI: 10.1200/JCO.2012.45.2615)

Phase III trial, $N = 636$, cT1N0, ER+, age ≥70 randomized to lumpectomy + tamoxifen versus lumpectomy + whole breast radiation + tamoxifen. Although whole breast radiation improved IBTR (2% vs. 9%), there was no difference in mastectomy rates, distant disease-free or breast cancer specific survival at 10 years.

### ASTRO Consensus Statement on Accelerated Partial Breast Irradiation (APBI) (Smith et al., *Int J Radiat Oncol Biol Phys* 2009; DOI: 10.1016/j.ijrobp.2009.02.031)

Systematic review and consensus statement of the appropriateness of APBI. Suitable: age >60, BRCA (–), invasive ductal, stage pT1N0 (with nodal evaluation), ER+, unicentric/focal disease, no lymphovascular space invasion (LVSI). Cautionary: age 50 to 59, stage pT2, ER–, with close margins (<2 mm), DCIS <3 cm. Unsuitable: age <50, pure DCIS >3 cm, who have not undergone SLNB or axillary dissection.

# 20: LOCALLY ADVANCED BREAST CANCER

*Adam Kole, MD, PhD*
*Sanjay Aneja, MD*
*Meena Moran, MD*

## WORKUP

### All Cases
- See Early Stage Breast Cancer chapter
- Axilla should be clinically and radiographically assessed
- U.S.-guided biopsy of any suspicious lymph nodes
- Can consider sentinel lymph node biopsy (SNLBx) for neo-adjuvant chemotherapy patients, alternatively, SNLBx can be performed after neo-adjuvant chemotherapy for initially occult or cN0 patients.
- Consider labs (CBC, LFTs, alk phos, etc.) and metastatic workup (chest CT, bone scan, PET/CT) for clinical stage IIIA (T3, N1) or greater, or as directed by signs/symptoms.

## TREATMENT RECOMMENDATIONS BY STAGE

| IIB (T3N0) – IIIC | Chemo → surgery (mastectomy or BCS) → RT<br>OR Surgery (mastectomy or BCS) → chemo → RT<br>Endocrine therapy for ER/PR + as indicated |
|---|---|
| T4d (inflammatory) | Chemo → response → modified radical mastectomy → RT<br>Chemo → no response → additional chemotherapy or RT → modified radical mastectomy → RT if not given pre-op |
| IV (metastatic) | Palliative endocrine therapy or chemotherapy<br>Antiosteoporosis therapy if bone metastases present<br>RT targeting symptomatic sites requiring palliation |

## National Comprehensive Cancer Network Contraindications to Breast-Conservation With RT

### Absolute
Pregnancy, diffuse microcalcifications suspicious for malignancy, inability to achieve good cosmesis (large tumor relative to breast size)

*Relative*

Prior ipsilateral RT, scleroderma/lupus, T3 tumors, genetic predisposition to breast cancer

## National Comprehensive Cancer Network Preferred Chemotherapy Regimens

*Her2-Negative Disease*

- Dose-dense adriamycin (ddAC, cyclophosphamide) × 4 cycles (q2 weeks) followed by T (paclitaxel) × 4 cycles (q2 weeks)
- ddAC × 4 cycles (q2 weeks) followed by T (lower dose) × 12 cycles (q1 week)
- TC (docetaxel and cyclophosphamide) × 4 cycles (q3 weeks)

*Her2-Positive Disease*

- AC or ddAC × 4 cycles (q2 or q3 weeks) followed by T (12 cycles q1 week or 4 cycles q2 weeks) with H (trastuzumab) × 12 cycles (q1 week). Trastuzumab continued q1 or q3 weeks for 1 year. Consider pertuzumab × 4 cycles (q3 weeks) during concurrent TH chemotherapy.
- TCH (docetaxel, carboplatin, trastuzumab) × 6 cycles (q3 weeks). Consider pertuzumab × 6 cycles (q3 weeks).

## TECHNICAL CONSIDERATIONS

### Simulation

Supine position, arms up, clinical breast borders and surgical scar wired (and drainage sites for inflammatory cases).

Technical considerations for decreasing lung and/or heart dose:

- Heart block (ensure breast tissue at risk is not blocked)
- Deep inspiration breath-hold
- Techniques that combine photons to decrease the impact of more penetrating photon beams

### Doses and Specifications (Post Mastectomy Radiation)

- Chestwall: 50 to 50.4 Gy in 1.8 to 2 Gy/fx.
- Bolus: 0.5 to 1.0 cm placed on chest wall for first 20 Gy, or every other day of treatment, or until brisk skin reaction occurs. Consider bolus for entire course of RT for inflammatory.
- Supraclavicular fossa: 46 to 50.4 Gy in 1.8 to 2 Gy/fx.

- Boost: 10 to 16 Gy in 2 Gy/fx. Typically 2 to 4 cm around the mastectomy scar treated with electrons ± bolus.
- Axilla: 46 to 50.4 Gy in 1.8 to 2 Gy/fx. Typically included as a component of chest wall and/or supraclavicular field. "Posterior axillary boost" can be added for larger patients to increase dose to mid-depth.

## Target Delineation

Contour normal structures (i.e., bilateral lungs, heart)

- CTV = as defined by a combination of Radiation Therapy Oncology Group (RTOG) Consensus Breast Cancer Atlas, clinical assessment of disease at risk and radiographic findings. Should include mastectomy scar and, for inflammatory breast cancer, drainage sites.
- Regional nodal CTV = Supraclavicular nodes, axilla (levels I–III) and internal mammary, when appropriate
- PTV = Breast/Chest wall CTV + 7-mm expansion (excludes heart and does not cross midline).
- PTV Eval = Subtracts PTV extending into lung (or chest wall for breast-conserving cases) and 3 to 5 mm off of skin anteriorly (build-up region)

## Treatment Planning

Breast-conserving therapy: 6 to 18 MV photons (often used in combination)

Tangential fields with forward planned or inverse planned segments to achieve **treatment goals/constraints**:

- **Cardiac:** $V_{\geq 20\,Gy} \leq 5\%$; $V_{\geq 10\,Gy} \leq 0\%$; Heart Dose$_{Mean}$: <400 cGy
- **Lung:** $V_{20Gy} < 15\%$, $V_{10\,Gy} < 35\%$
- **Whole breast PTV Eval:** $V_{\geq 95\%} \geq 95\%$; Max dose <115%, $V_{108\%} \leq 50\%$.

Postmastectomy radiation therapy: Can be more complex than treatment to intact breast due to inherent anatomic challenges associated with the reconstructed chest wall and more routine inclusion of regional nodes, which can make dose constraints more onerous to respect.

Common methods for inclusion of internal mammary nodes:

1. Deep tangents
2. Photon–electron or electron-alone internal mammary fields matched to photon tangents

## SELECTED STUDIES

### Danish 82b and 82c Trials (Nielsen, *J Clin Oncol* 2006; DOI: 10.1200/JCO.2005.02.8738)

Long-term (18-year) follow-up of 3,083 patients randomized to adjuvant chemotherapy and post-mastectomy radiation versus adjuvant chemotherapy alone. Post-mastectomy radiation reduced loco-regional recurrences from 49% to 14% and rate of distant metastases from 64% to 53%, with prior studies showing ~10% survival benefit with post-mastectomy radiation.

### British Columbia Post-Mastectomy Radiation Trial (Ragaz, *J Natl Cancer Inst* 2005)

Long-term (20-year) follow-up of 318 patients randomized to adjuvant chemotherapy and post-mastectomy radiation versus adjuvant chemotherapy alone. Post-mastectomy radiation reduced locoregional recurrences from 26% to 10%, improved breast cancer-specific survival from 38% to 53%, and improved overall survival from 37% to 47%.

### Early Breast Cancer Trialists' Collaborative Group Meta-Analysis (EBCTCG, *Lancet* 2014; DOI: 10.1016/S0140-6736(14)60488-8)

The 20-year follow-up of the meta-analysis of patients treated on the post-mastectomy radiation trials. Among 1,314 women with 1 to 3 positive lymph nodes, breast cancer mortality is improved from 50.2% to 42.3% with post-mastectomy radiation; whereas among 1,772 women with 4+ positive lymph nodes, post-mastectomy radiation improves breast cancer mortality from 80.0% to 70.7%.

### Review of National Surgical Adjuvant Breast and Bowel Project Trials (Taghian, *J Clin Oncol* 2004; DOI: 10.1200/JCO.2004.01.042)

Assessed patterns of locoregional failure in lymph node-positive 5,758 patients enrolled onto multiple National Surgical Adjuvant Breast and Bowel Project trials and treated with mastectomy, adjuvant chemotherapy, and without post-mastectomy radiation. Chest wall and mastectomy scar recurrences were most common (57%), followed by supraclavicular lymph node recurrences (23%), and axillary (12%). Predictors for locoregional failure as a first event included age, tumor size, premenopausal status, number of positive lymph nodes, and number of lymph nodes excised at dissection.

## AMAROS Trial (Donker, *Lancet Oncol* 2014; DOI: 10.1016/S1470-2045(14)70460-7)

Five-year outcomes of 4,806 patients with cT1-2 cN0 disease to receive either a surgical axillary lymph node dissection (ALND) or axillary RT to levels I to III and medial supraclavicular fossa, in the event of positive sentinel lymph node. Five-year axillary recurrence rates were not significantly different, with 0.43% in the ALND group and 1.19% in the axillary RT group. Rates of lymphedema were worse in those undergoing ALND.

## European Organisation for Research and Treatment of Cancer Nodal Irradiation Trial (Poortmans, *N Engl J Med* 2015; DOI: 10.1056/NEJMoa1415369)

Ten-year outcomes of 4,004 stage I–III patients with medial/central tumors or node (+) disease receiving whole breast RT or post-mastectomy radiation, randomized to regional nodal RT (directed to the axilla, supraclavicular fossa, and IM nodes) versus no regional nodal RT. The 10-year distant disease-free survival and disease-free survival were improved with regional nodal RT. Overall survival showed a nonsignificant trend favoring comprehensive nodal RT, with 10-year survival of 82.3% with nodal RT versus 80.7% without.

## MA-20 Nodal Irradiation Trial (Whelan, *N Engl J Med* 2015; DOI: 10.1056/NEJMoa1415340)

Ten-year outcomes of 1,832 patients with pN+ disease or pN0 with high-risk features receiving whole breast RT or post-mastectomy radiation, randomized to regional nodal RT (directed to the axilla, supraclavicular fossa, and IM nodes) versus no regional nodal RT, (similar to European Organisation for Research and Treatment of Cancer (EORTC) trial noted previously). Disease-free survival, but not overall survival, was improved in the regional nodal RT group. Rates of pneumonitis and lymphedema were high in patients receiving nodal RT.

# 21: ESOPHAGEAL CANCER

*Charles Rutter, MD*
*Kimberly Lauren Johung, MD, PhD*

## WORKUP

### All Cases

- H&P (dysphagia, weight loss, performance status)
- Esophagogastroduodenoscopy (EGD) with biopsy (human epidermal growth factor receptor 2 [HER2] testing if adenocarcinoma)
- Endoscopic ultrasound (evaluates depth of invasion, nodes)
- CT chest/abdomen with PO and IV contrast
- PET/CT
- Bronchoscopy (if at/above carina)
- Counseling on nutrition and smoking cessation
- Consider gastrostomy tube for nutrition if obstructed

## TREATMENT RECOMMENDATIONS BY STAGE

| | |
|---|---|
| Tis/T1aN0 | Endoscopic resection ± ablation OR Esophagectomy |
| T1bN0 Operable | Esophagectomy |
| T1bN0 Inoperable or Cervical Esophagus | Definitive chemoRT |
| T1bN+ or T2-T4aN0-N+ and Operable | Neoadjuvant chemoRT → Esophagectomy |
| T1bN+ or T2-T4aN0-N+ and Inoperable or Cervical Esophagus | Definitive chemoRT |
| T4b AnyN, M0 | Definitive chemoRT |
| M1 | Systemic therapy ± palliative RT or palliative/supportive care |
| pT3-T4, pN+, or positive margins | Post-op chemoRT (if no neoadjuvant RT was delivered) |

## TECHNICAL CONSIDERATIONS

### Simulation

- Simulate supine with custom immobilization
- Assessment and management of respiratory motion (e.g., 4DCT + ITV, gating)

**Dose Prescription**

*Definitive ChemoRT*
- 45 Gy in 1.8 Gy/fx to esophagus and elective regional nodes
- Sequential boost to primary tumor and involved nodes to 50.4 Gy in 1.8 Gy/fx or
- Dose painted IMRT with 45 Gy in 1.8 Gy/fx to esophagus and elective regional nodes; 50 Gy in 2 Gy/fx to primary tumor and involved nodes

*Pre-Op ChemoRT*
- 41.4 to 50.4 Gy in 1.8 Gy/fx to esophagus and elective regional nodes
- Sequential boost to primary tumor and involved nodes to 50.4 Gy in 1.8 Gy/fx or
- Dose painted IMRT as noted previously for definitive chemoRT

*Post-Op RT*
- 45 to 50.4 Gy in 1.8 to 2 Gy/fx

**Target Delineation**

Contour on soft tissue windows

See Expert Consensus contouring guidelines for IMRT (Wu, *IJROBP* 2015; DOI: 10.1016/j.ijrobp.2015.03.030)
- GTV = Gross tumor and involved nodes based on EGD and imaging
- ITV = GTV contoured throughout respiratory cycle
- CTV = ITV + 3.5-cm to 4-cm superior and inferior expansion along the esophagus and 1-cm radial expansion; consider elective treatment of bilateral supraclavicular and mediastinal nodes for tumors above the carina and celiac and gastrohepatic nodes for tumors below the carina
- PTV = CTV + 0.5 cm using daily IGRT

**Treatment Planning**
- 3DCRT or IMRT
- 6-MV to 10-MV photons
- Use heterogeneity corrections

**FOLLOW UP**

If asymptomatic: H&P every 3 to 6 months × 2 years, then every 6 to 12 months × 3 years, then annually. Imaging and EGD as clinically indicated.

**SELECTED STUDIES**

### Cancer and Leukemia Group B (CALGB) 9781 (Tepper, *J Clin Oncol* 2008; DOI: 10.1200/JCO.2007.12.9593)

Modern trial comparing surgery alone to neoadjuvant chemoRT to 50.4 Gy with Cisplatin/Fluorouracil (5-FU), followed by surgery in T1-3N0-1 patients (75% adenocarcinoma). At 5 years, neoadjuvant chemoRT improved overall survival (OS) (39% vs. 16%) and progression-free survival (PFS) (28% vs. 15%), without operative mortality in the neoadjuvant therapy arm.

### CROSS Trial (Shapiro, *Lancet Oncol* 2015 Long-Term Results; DOI: 10.1016/S1470-2045(15)00040-6)

A second modern trial of surgery ± neoadjuvant chemoRT. The chemoRT regimen used lower RT doses (41.4 Gy in 1.8 Gy fractions) and different chemotherapy (weekly Carboplatin/Paclitaxel), but still demonstrated improved OS (47% vs. 33% at 5 years, median 48.6 vs. 24.0 months), PFS, locoregional and distant control, and greater margin-negative resection rates in a population of patients with T1N1 or T2-3N0-1 disease, predominantly (80%) of the distal esophagus/gastroesophageal (GE) junction.

### German Trial (Stahl, *J Clin Oncol* 2005; DOI: 10.1200/JCO.2005.00.034)

Compared trimodality therapy (chemoRT + surgery) to definitive chemoRT in a cohort of patients with T3-4N0-1 squamous cell carcinoma of the esophagus. Both arms received three cycles of induction Cisplatin/5-FU/Etoposide before undergoing Cisplatin/Etoposide × one cycle + 40 Gy RT then surgery (trimodality arm) versus Cisplatin/Etoposide × one cycle + 64 to 65 Gy RT (definitive arm). There was no difference in OS with the addition of surgery (40% vs. 35% at 2 years), although cancer-specific survival and local control were improved in the trimodality arm.

### RTOG 8501 (Cooper, *JAMA* 1999; DOI: 10.1001/jama.281.17.1623; Herskovic, *N Engl J Med* 1992; DOI: 10.1056/NEJM199206113262403)

Trial of definitive RT versus definitive chemoRT among patients with nonmetastatic thoracic esophageal cancer (88% squamous cell carcinoma). On the chemoRT arm, four cycles of Cisplatin/5-FU were given concurrently with RT to 50 Gy, while the RT-alone arm received 64 Gy. ChemoRT improved OS at 5 years (26% vs. 0%), as well as local and distant control, compared to patients treated with RT alone. Importantly, there were no long-term survivors on the RT-alone arm, underscoring the fact that definitive RT alone has no role in curative-intent therapy.

### Intergroup 0123 (Minsky, *J Clin Oncol* 2002; DOI: 10.1200/JCO.20.5.1167)

Comparison of standard-dose (50.4 Gy) versus dose-escalated (64.8 Gy) Cisplatin/5-FU chemoRT in T1-4N0-1 esophageal cancer. Dose-escalation achieved using 14.4 Gy boost to GTV + 2 cm after initial 50.4 Gy. There were no differences in OS or control at locoregional or distant sites between arms, and there were more treatment-related deaths on the dose-escalated arm (11 vs. 2), although the majority of these deaths (7 of 11) occurred before 50.4 Gy.

### Contouring Guidelines (Wu, *Int J Radiat Oncol Biol Phys* 2015; DOI: 10.1016/j.ijrobp.2015.03.030)

Expert consensus contouring guidelines for IMRT in esophageal and GE junction cancer.

### 3DCRT versus IMRT Comparison (Lin, *Int J Radiat Oncol Biol Phys* 2012; DOI: 10.1016/j.ijrobp.2012.02.015)

Propensity score-based comparison of long-term outcomes with 3DCRT versus IMRT for esophageal cancer.

# 22: GASTRIC CANCER

*Charles Rutter, MD*
*Kimberly Lauren Johung, MD, PhD*

## WORKUP

### All Cases

- H&P (early satiety, weight loss, performance status)
- Esophagogastroduodenoscopy (EGD) with biopsy (with human epidermal growth factor receptor 2 [HER2] testing)
- Endoscopic ultrasound (depth of invasion, nodes)
- CT C/A/P with PO and IV contrast
- Consider PET/CT
- Counseling on smoking cessation and nutrition

## TREATMENT RECOMMENDATIONS BY STAGE

| | |
|---|---|
| Tis/T1a Operable | Endoscopic resection OR Gastrectomy |
| Tis/T1a Inoperable | Endoscopic resection |
| T1bN0 Operable | Gastrectomy |
| T2-T4bN0-N+ Operable | Gastrectomy OR Chemo → Gastrectomy → Chemo OR Chemoradiation → Gastrectomy |
| T1b-T4bN0-N+ Inoperable | Definitive chemoradiaton ± Gastrectomy if conversion to operable |
| pT2N0 after gastrectomy alone | Adjuvant chemoradiation, chemotherapy, or observation |
| pT3-4N0 or any N+ after gastrectomy alone | Adjuvant chemoradiation or chemotherapy |
| pT3-4N0 or any N+ after neoadjuvant therapy + gastrectomy | Adjuvant chemotherapy |
| Positive surgical margins | Adjuvant chemoradiation (if not given preoperatively) |
| Metastatic | Systemic therapy, palliative care |

Gastrectomy may be distal, subtotal, or total depending on location; for T4 lesions, en bloc resection of invaded structures; nodal dissection to include perigastric nodes (D1) and often nodes along named vessels (left gastric, hepatic, splenic, celiac) of celiac axis (D2) with total of at least 15 nodes.

## TECHNICAL CONSIDERATIONS

### Simulation
- Simulate supine with custom immobilization
- Nothing by mouth (NPO) 3 hours before simulation and treatment
- PO contrast
- Assessment and management of respiratory motion (e.g. 4DCT + ITV, gating)

### Dose Prescription
- Adjuvant chemoRT: 45 Gy in 1.8 Gy/fx;
- If microscopic residual disease boost 5.4 Gy in 1.8 Gy/fx (50.4 Gy total)
- If gross residual disease boost 9 Gy in 1.8 Gy/fx (54 Gy total)
- Neoadjuvant chemoRT: 45 to 50.4 Gy in 1.8 Gy/fx
- Definitive chemoRT: 45 Gy in 1.8 Gy/fx; boost tumor to 50.4 to 54 Gy in 1.8 Gy/fx

### Target Delineation
*Contour on Soft Tissue Windows*
- GTV = gross tumor based on EGD, endoscopic ultrasound (EUS), and imaging
- ITV = GTV contoured throughout respiratory cycle
- CTV = Tumor bed (merge pre-op imaging and use surgical clips), anastomoses, and most often the gastric remnant
  - **Primary in Proximal Third/Cardia**
  - 3- to 5-cm of distal esophagus
  - Nodes: perigastric, celiac, splenic hilum, porta hepatis
  - **Primary in Middle Third/Body**
  - Nodes: perigastric, suprapancreatic, celiac, splenic hilum, porta hepatis, pancreaticoduodenal
  - **Primary in Distal Third/Antrum and Pylorus**
  - First and second portion of duodenum if tumor extends to gastroduodenal junction
  - Nodes: perigastric, suprapancreatic, celiac, porta hepatis, pancreaticoduodenal
- PTV = 0.5- to 1-cm expansion on CTV based on institutional practice and use of daily image-guided radiation therapy (IGRT)

### Treatment Planning
- IMRT or three-dimensional conformal radiotherapy
- 6- to 10-MV photons
- Heterogeneity corrections

## FOLLOW UP

If asymptomatic: H&P every 3 to 6 months × 1 to 2 years, then every 6 to 12 months × 3 years, then annually. Imaging, EGD, and labs as indicated.

## SELECTED STUDIES

### Intergroup 0116 (MacDonald, *N Engl J Med* 2001; DOI: 10.1056/NEJMoa010187; Update *J Clin Oncol* 2012; DOI: 10.1200/JCO.2012.42.4069)

Randomized patients with T2-4N0 or any N+ gastric or gastro-esophageal (GE) junction cancer to surgery ± adjuvant chemoRT to 45 Gy with Fluorouracil (5-FU)/leukovorin. Most patients had ≤ D1 nodal dissection. At 10 years median follow-up, adjuvant chemoRT improved overall survival (OS) (median 35 vs. 27 months) and relapse-free survival (RFS) (median 27 vs. 19 months).

### MAGIC Trial (Cunningham, *N Engl J Med* 2006; DOI: 10.1056/NEJMoa055531)

Compared surgery ± perioperative Epirubicin/Cisplatin/5-FU (ECF) chemotherapy (three cycles pre- and three cycles postoperatively) in patients with stage II or higher gastric, GE junction, or distal esophageal cancer (75% gastric). Type of surgery and extent of nodal dissection left to surgeon discretion (slightly greater D2 than D1 dissection). Perioperative ECF led to improved OS (36% vs. 23% at 5 years), progression-free survival (PFS), and better surgical outcomes compared to surgery alone.

### ARTIST Trial (Park, *J Clin Oncol* 2015; DOI: 10.1200/JCO.2014.58.3930)

Patients with stage IB-IVA gastric cancer s/p gastrectomy with D2 nodal dissection were randomized to post-op capecitabine/cisplatin (XP) × six cycles versus XP × two cycles followed by chemoRT to 45 Gy with capecitabine and XP × two cycles. At 7 years median follow-up, chemoRT did not improve disease-free survival (DFS) or OS overall, though on subgroup analysis, 3-year DFS was improved in node-positive patients (76% vs. 72%) and intestinal type gastric cancer (94% vs. 83%).

## Dutch Nodal Dissection Trial (Bonenkamp, *N Engl J Med* 1999; DOI: 10.1056/NEJM199903253401210)

To address the controversy regarding the optimal extent of node dissection, this trial randomized patients to D1 versus D2 node dissection (performed under the supervision of expert Japanese surgeons). No adjuvant therapies were allowed. The results demonstrated no difference in OS or RFS between D1 and D2 dissection, but higher toxicity (including greater in-hospital mortality) following D2 dissection.

## ToGA Trial (Bang, *Lancet Oncol* 2010; DOI: 10.1016/S0140-6736(10)61121-X)

Patients with advanced (97% metastatic) HER2+ gastric or GE junction adenocarcinoma were randomized to Cisplatin/5-FU or Cisplatin/Capecitabine ± Trastuzumab for six cycles. The addition of Trastuzumab led to an improvement in OS (median 14 vs. 11 months), PFS, and response rate and duration. The benefit of Trastuzumab was strongest for fluorescence in situ hybridization (FISH+) or immunohistochemistry (IHC) 2 to 3+ results.

# 23: HEPATOBILIARY

*Charles Rutter, MD*
*Kimberly Lauren Johung, MD, PhD*

## WORKUP

### All Cases

- H&P (alcoholism, hepatitis, family hx, abdominal exam)
- Abdominal ultrasound
- Abdominal MRI or CT with intravenous (IV) contrast (three phase for hepatocellular carcinoma [HCC])
- Chest CT
- Bone scan as clinically indicated for HCC
- Alpha-fetoprotein (AFP), carcinoembryonic antigen (CEA), cancer antigen 19-9, hepatitis panel
- Standard labs, including liver function tests (LFTs) and coagulation panel
- Core biopsy or fine-needle aspiration (FNA) to confirm HCC if <2 classic enhancements by CT or MRI
- Surgical consultation
- Consider staging laparoscopy for cholangiocarcinoma or gallbladder cancer
- Consider cholangiography (such as magnetic resonance cholangiopancreatography [MRCP]) for extrahepatic cholangiocarcinoma or gallbladder cancer

## TREATMENT RECOMMENDATIONS BY STAGE

| Hepatocellular carcinoma | |
|---|---|
| Potentially resectable | Resection<br>OR transplant ± local therapy to bridge to transplant (Locoregional therapy: ablation, e.g., radiofrequency or cryoablation), stereotactic body radiation therapy (SBRT), or arterially delivered treatments (e.g., transarterial chemoembolization [TACE] or radioembolization with yttrium-90 microspheres) |
| Unresectable | Transplant<br>OR locoregional therapy vs. systemic therapy (usually sorafenib)<br>OR clinical trial<br>OR supportive care |

(continued)

*(continued)*

| Localized but medically inoperable | Locoregional therapy OR systemic therapy (sorafenib) OR supportive care OR clinical trial |
|---|---|
| Metastatic | Systemic therapy (sorafenib) OR clinical trial OR supportive care |

**Gallbladder cancer**

| Resectable | Radical cholecystectomy with en bloc adjacent hepatic resection, lymphadenectomy, ± bile duct excision → Consider adjuvant 5-FU-based chemoRT vs. systemic therapy |
|---|---|
| Incidental finding on simple cholecystectomy | Stage, then if localized pT1b or greater: hepatic resection, lymphadenectomy, ± bile duct excision vs. treatment per unresectable paradigm if further surgery feasible → Consider adjuvant 5-FU-based chemoRT vs. systemic therapy |
| Unresectable | Systemic therapy (usually gemcitabine/cisplatin) ± 5-FU-based chemoRT vs. supportive care vs. clinical trial |
| Metastatic | Consider palliative biliary drainage Systemic therapy OR supportive care OR clinical trial |

**Intrahepatic cholangiocarcinoma**

| Resectable | Resection → ± adjuvant chemotherapy (if R0 resection) vs. chemoRT (if R1 resection) |
|---|---|
| Unresectable | Combination chemotherapy (usually gemcitabine/cisplatin) OR 5-FU-based chemoRT OR clinical trial OR locoregional therapy OR supportive care |
| Metastatic | Combination chemotherapy OR clinical trial OR locoregional therapy OR supportive care |

**Extrahepatic cholangiocarcinoma (EHC)**

| Resectable | Resection (± pre-op biliary drainage) → 5-FU-based chemoRT (for R0–R1 N0) vs. 5-FU or gemcitabine-based chemotherapy alone (for R0–R2 or N+) |
|---|---|

*(continued)*

*(continued)*

| Unresectable | Combination chemotherapy (usually gemcitabine/cisplatin) OR 5-FU-based chemoRT OR clinical trial OR supportive care Consider biliary drainage as indicated |
| Metastatic | Combination chemotherapy OR clinical trial OR supportive care |

Cautious patient selection for SBRT is required because baseline liver dysfunction is common in this population. Childs Pugh scores should be calculated. Much of the safety data regarding external beam radiation therapy (EBRT) for HCC in particular originates from patients with Childs Pugh A liver disease.

## TECHNICAL CONSIDERATIONS

### Simulation
- Simulate supine with custom immobilization
- Assessment and management of respiratory motion (e.g., 4DCT + ITV, gating, and abdominal compression especially for SBRT)
- PO contrast, consider IV contrast arterial and venous phase scans

### Dose Prescription
*Hepatocellular Carcinoma*
- SBRT in 3 to 5 fractions to highest dose achievable while respecting normal tissue constraints

*Biliary Cancers*
- 45 Gy in 1.8 Gy/fx, to regional nodes and tumor/tumor bed then boost tumor/tumor bed to and 50 to 59.4 Gy in 1.8 Gy/fx, or intraluminal brachytherapy boost
- Consider SBRT for intrahepatic cholangiocarcinoma with dosing as per HCC

### Target Delineation
*Hepatocellular Carcinoma*
- GTV = both parenchymal and vascular disease as seen on CT or MRI, often hyperintense on arterial phase and hypointense on venous phase IV contrast scans

- ITV = GTV contoured throughout respiratory cycle
- CTV = often no expansion from GTV to CTV for SBRT
- PTV = CTV + 4 to 10 mm, depending on method of respiratory motion management and daily image guidance

*Biliary Cancers*
- GTV = gross tumor as seen on CT or MRI; fuse pre-op imaging to define tumor bed for adjuvant treatment
- CTV = 0.5- to 1.0-cm margin on GTV for microscopic disease; regional nodes (porta hepatis, celiac, pancreaticoduodenal)
- PTV = 0.5- to 1-cm expansion on CTV based upon institutional practice and use of daily IGRT

**Treatment Planning**
- IMRT versus 3DCRT versus SBRT
- 6- to 10-MV photons
- Use heterogeneity corrections

**FOLLOW UP**

If asymptomatic: Imaging and tumor markers every 3 to 6 months × 2 years, then every 6 to 12 months

**SELECTED STUDIES**

**University of Toronto SBRT (Tse, *J Clin Oncol* 2008; DOI: 10.1200/JCO.2007.14.3529)**
In this phase I study, 41 patients with unresectable HCC or intra-hepatic cholangiocarcinoma were treated with 6-fraction SBRT to a mean of 36 Gy (range 24–54 Gy, escalated based upon effective dose to the uninvolved liver). Local control was obtained in 65% at 1 year, median survival was 13.4 months, and toxicity was acceptable, with no grade 4 to 5 toxicity observed.

**Phase I and II Trials of SBRT for HCC (Bujold, *J Clin Oncol* 2013; DOI: 10.1200/JCO.2012.48.2703)**
Patients with HCC and Childs Pugh A liver scores who were unsuitable for surgery, TACE, radiofrequency ablation (RFA), or alcohol ablation were treated with SBRT from 24 to 54 Gy in 6 fractions. Toxicity ≥ grade 3 occurred in 30% of patients. Local control at 1 year was 87%.

### Phase II Trial of SBRT After TACE (Kang, *Cancer* 2012; DOI: 10.1002/cncr.27533)

In this phase II trial, 47 evaluable patients were treated with 3-fraction SBRT to a median of 57 Gy (range 42–60 Gy) following incomplete response to 1 to 5 sessions of TACE. Complete responses were observed in approximately 38%, and local control and overall survival (OS) at 2 years were 95% and 69%, respectively.

### TACE Plus Radiation Therapy versus TACE Alone for HCC (Huo, JAMA 2015; DOI: 10.1001/jamaoncol.2015.2189)

Meta-analysis of 25 trials including 2,577 patients with unresectable HCC comparing the safety and efficacy of TACE plus RT versus TACE alone. RT was a mix of conventional fractionation, hypofractionation, and hyperfractionation to a BED of 30.6 to 100.8 Gy using 3D conformal or stereotactic techniques. Though adverse effects including gastroduodenal ulcers, elevated alanine transaminase (ALT), and elevated total bilirubin were increased with TACE plus RT versus TACE alone, TACE plus RT was associated with improved complete response and OS.

### SBRT versus RFA for HCC (Wahl, *J Clin Oncol* 2015; DOI: 10.1200/JCO.2015.61.4925)

Retrospective single institution analysis of 224 patients with inoperable HCC treated with RFA versus SBRT. Freedom from local progression (FFLP) was 83.6% with RFA and 97.4% with SBRT at 1 year, and 80.2% with RFA and 83.8% with SBRT at 2 years. FFLP was significantly decreased with RFA versus SBRT for tumors $\geq 2$ cm (HR 3.35, $P = .025$). One-year OS was 70% with RFA and 74% with SBRT. Rates of acute grade 3 or higher toxicity were not significantly different.

### Hypofractionated RT for Unresectable HCC or Intrahepatic Cholangiocarcinoma (Hong, *J Clin Oncol* 2016; DOI: 10.1200/JCO.2015.64.2710)

Phase II multi-institutional study of 92 patients with unresectable HCC or intrahepatic cholangiocarcinoma and Childs Pugh A or B scores were treated with hypofractionated proton beam therapy in 15 fractions to a median dose of 58 Gy. Toxicity was low (4.8% grade 3, and no grade 4 or 5 reported). Local control at 2 years was 95% for HCC and 94% for intrahepatic cholangiocarcinoma, and OS at 2 years was 63% for HCC and 47% for intrahepatic cholangiocarcinoma.

### Meta-Analysis of Adjuvant Therapy for Biliary Cancers (Horgan, *J Clin Oncol* 2012; DOI: 10.1200/JCO.2011.40.5381)

Meta-analysis of 22 studies including 6,712 patients who underwent curative-intent surgery for biliary tract cancers (mostly extrahepatic cholangiocarcinoma or gallbladder cancers; only one study included intrahepatic cholangiocarcinoma). Adjuvant therapy was associated with the greatest survival benefit in patients with node positive disease or R1 resections. The majority of node positive patients received chemotherapy alone. Two thirds of R1 patients received adjuvant radiation and a benefit was seen with RT for all disease sites.

### SWOG S0809 (Ben-Josef, *J Clin Oncol* 2015; DOI: 10.1200/JCO.2014.60.2219)

Patients with T2 to T4 or N+ extrahepatic cholangiocarcinoma or gallbladder carcinoma were treated with adjuvant gemcitabine/capecitabine × four cycles followed by chemoRT (45 Gy to regional nodes and 54–59.4 Gy to tumor bed with concurrent capecitabine). Median OS was 35 months, and 2-year OS was 65%. The regimen was tolerable with promising efficacy.

# 24: PANCREATIC CANCER

*Charles Rutter, MD*
*Kimberly Lauren Johung, MD, PhD*

## WORKUP

### All Cases

- H&P (weight loss, performance status, jaundice)
- CT Abdomen/pelvis using pancreas protocol
- Endoscopic retrograde cholangiopancreatography (ERCP) and/or endoscopic ultrasound (EUS) with biopsy
- Chest CT
- Consider PET/CT
- CA 19–9
- Consider staging laparoscopy before definitive resection
- Consider placement of metal biliary stent if jaundiced

## TREATMENT RECOMMENDATIONS BY STAGE

| Resectable | Surgery → Chemo<br>OR Surgery → chemoRT → chemo<br>OR Surgery → chemo → chemoRT |
|---|---|
| Borderline Resectable | Chemo ± chemoRT → surgery (if conversion to resectable)<br>If resected consider further adjuvant chemotherapy |
| Unresectable | Chemotherapy<br>OR chemo → ChemoRT if good performance status and no distant mets |
| Metastatic | Chemotherapy, palliative care |

### National Comprehensive Cancer Network Resectability Criteria (2015)

- **Resectable**—M0; no contact with celiac axis (CA), superior mesenteric artery (SMA), or common hepatic artery (CHA); ≤180° contact with superior mesenteric vein (SMV) or portal vein (PV) without vein contour irregularity
- **Borderline Resectable**—M0; ≤180° contact with SMA; common hepatic involvement not extending to CA; ≤180° contact with CA for body/tail tumors; >180° contact with SMV or PV and/or contour irregularity or thrombosis amenable to vein reconstruction; inferior vena cava (IVC) involvement

- **Unresectable**—M1; >180° contact with CA or SMA; aortic involvement; SMV or PV involvement or occlusion not amenable to vein reconstruction
- *Resection may consist of a pancreaticoduodenectomy (Whipple) or distal pancreatectomy

## TECHNICAL CONSIDERATIONS

### Simulation
- Simulate supine with custom immobilization
- Assessment and management of respiratory motion (e.g., 4DCT + ITV, gating) PO contrast, consider IV contrast

### Dose Prescription
- Definitive chemoRT: 50 to 54 Gy in 1.8 to 2 Gy/fx
- Neoadjuvant chemoRT: 50 to 54 Gy in 1.8 to 2 Gy/fx
- Adjuvant chemoRT: 50.4 Gy in 1.8 Gy/fx

### Target Delineation
Contour on soft tissue windows

- GTV = primary tumor + positive nodes (fluorodeoxyglucose [FDG]-avid or size >1 cm) based on imaging and EUS findings
- ITV = GTV contoured throughout respiratory cycle
- CTV =
  - Adjuvant:
    - Tumor bed (based on pre-op imaging, surgical clips, operative and pathology reports); Anastomoses (pancreaticojejunostomy, choledochal or hepaticojejunostomy); Regional nodes (peripancreatic, celiac, superior mesenteric, porta hepatis, and para-aortic)
  - Neoadjuvant or definitive:
    - 0.5- to 1.5-cm margin on GTV for microscopic disease
- PTV = 0.5- to 1-cm expansion on CTV based on institutional practice and use of daily image-guided radiation therapy (IGRT).

### Treatment Planning
- IMRT or 3D
- 6- to 10-MV photons
- Use heterogeneity corrections

## FOLLOW UP

If asymptomatic: H&P, CA 19 to -9 level, and CT A/P per pancreas protocol q3 to 6 months × 2 years, q6 to 12 months × 3 years, then annually

## SELECTED STUDIES

### Gastrointestinal Tumor Study Group 9173 (Kalser, *Arch Surg* 1985; DOI: 10.1001/archsurg.1985.01390320023003)

Historical trial comparing adjuvant chemoRT (40 Gy in two split courses 2 weeks apart with bolus Fluorouracil [5-FU], followed by 2 years of weekly 5-FU) to observation following margin-negative resection. This study demonstrated that adjuvant chemoRT improved overall survival (OS) and progression-free survival (PFS), despite the split-course radiation therapy (RT) regimen.

### European Study Group for Pancreatic Cancer-1 (Neoptolemos, *N Engl J Med* 2004; DOI: 10.1056/NEJMoa032295)

Patients with resected pancreatic cancer were randomized (in a 2 × 2 schema) to observation, chemotherapy (5-FU/Leukovorin × six cycles), chemoRT (40 Gy split course with bolus 5-FU), or chemoRT followed by chemotherapy. The results demonstrated inferior survival on the chemoRT containing arms, and superior survival on the chemotherapy alone arms. However, these findings are confounded by uncertainties regarding treatment allotment and the antiquated chemoRT regimen used.

### Radiation Therapy Oncology Group 9704 (Regine, *Ann Surg Oncol* 2011 — Long-Term Results; DOI: 10.1245/s10434-011-1630-6)

A randomized comparison of gemcitabine versus 5-FU chemotherapy prior to and after 5-FU-based chemoRT to 50.4 Gy among patients with gross total resection of pancreatic cancer. Overall, the results demonstrated equivalence of the two regimens, although there was a trend toward improved survival with gemcitabine for pancreatic head tumors.

### CONKO-001 (Oettle, *JAMA* 2013 — Long-Term Results; DOI: 10.1001/jama.2013.279201)

This trial randomized patients after R0 or R1 resection of pancreatic cancer to adjuvant gemcitabine (× 6 cycles) versus observation. Adjuvant gemcitabine as compared to no adjuvant therapy improved median disease-free survival (13.4 vs. 6.7 months) and median OS (22.8 vs. 20.2 months).

### Eastern Cooperative Oncology Group 4201 (Loehrer, *J Clin Oncol* 2011; DOI: 10.1200/JCO.2011.34.8904)

Patients with locally advanced unresectable pancreatic adenocarcinoma were randomized to chemotherapy alone (gemcitabine weekly × 6) versus chemoRT (50.4 Gy + weekly dose-reduced gemcitabine) followed by consolidation with five cycles of gemcitabine. The trial closed early due to slow accrual, but still demonstrated an OS advantage to chemoRT, improving median survival from 9.2 to 11 months.

### GERCOR Retrospective (Huguet, *J Clin Oncol* 2007; DOI: 10.1200/JCO.2006.07.5663)

This combined analysis evaluated outcomes achieved by locally advanced pancreatic cancer patients treated on a variety of GERCOR randomized trials. Those without metastatic disease after a period of initial chemotherapy could receive chemoRT versus continuing chemotherapy at the investigator's discretion. Patients selected to receive chemoRT experienced improved OS (median 15 vs. 11.7 months) and PFS (median 10.8 vs. 7.4 months), emphasizing the role for chemoRT in locally advanced pancreatic cancer.

### FOLFIRINOX versus Gemcitabine (Conroy, *N Engl J Med* 2011; DOI: 10.1056/NEJMoa1011923)

An important trial that compared FOLFIRINOX (5-FU, Leukovorin, Irinotecan, Oxaliplatin) versus Gemcitabine in newly diagnosed metastatic pancreatic cancer patients. The results demonstrated superior OS (median 11.1 vs. 6.8 months), PFS (median 6.4 vs. 3.3 months), and response rate (32% vs. 9%) with FOLFIRINOX. These results have led to the utilization of this regimen in selected patients with locally advanced pancreatic cancer.

### Metastatic Pancreatic Adenocarcinoma Clinical Trial—nab-Paclitaxel Plus Gemcitabine versus Gemcitabine (Van Hoff, *N Engl J Med* 2013; DOI: 10.1056/NEJMoa1304369)

Patients with metastatic pancreatic cancer were randomized to nab-paclitaxel plus gemcitabine versus gemcitabine monotherapy. The combination of nab-paclitaxel plus gemcitabine demonstrated superior OS (median 8.5 vs. 6.7 months), PFS (median 5.5 vs. 3.7 months), and response rate (23% vs. 7%). Similar to the study of Conroy et al, these results have led to the use of nab-paclitaxel plus gemcitabine in selected patients with localized pancreatic cancer.

### Stereotactic Body Radiation Therapy Phase II Multi-Institutional Trial (Herman, *Cancer* 2015; DOI: 10.1002/cncr.29161)

Patients with locally advanced pancreatic cancer were treated with 3 weekly doses of gemcitabine followed by SBRT (33 Gy in 5 fractions) and gemcitabine until progression or limiting toxicity. Rates of acute and late gastrointestinal (GI) toxicity were 2% and 11%, respectively. Local control at 1 year was 78%, and median OS was 13.9 months. These results suggest that SBRT should be further investigated and considered for treatment as part of a clinical trial.

# 25: RECTAL CANCER

*Charles Rutter, MD*
*Kimberly Lauren Johung, MD, PhD*

## WORKUP

### All Cases
- H&P (family history, sphincter function, rectal exam)
- Colonoscopy with biopsy
- Anoscopy
- Transrectal ultrasound or MRI for T-staging
- CT chest/abdomen/pelvis
- Carcinoembryonic antigen (CEA)

## TREATMENT RECOMMENDATIONS BY STAGE

| | |
|---|---|
| cT1N0 | Transanal excision if favorable (≤3 cm, <30% circumference, well to moderately differentiated, no lymphovascular invasion (LVI), >3-mm margins) If upstaged to pT2 or positive margins, perform completion trans-abdominal resection OR trans-abdominal resection |
| cT2N0 | Trans-abdominal resection |
| pT3-4, pN+, or positive margin after primary surgery | Chemo (usually folinic acid, fluorouracil, and oxaliplatin (FOLFOX) × four cycles) → chemoRT (Capecitabine + RT) → further chemo (usually FOLFOX × four cycles) |
| cT3-4N0 or any N+ and/or medically inoperable | ChemoRT (± preceding induction chemotherapy) → trans-abdominal resection if resectable → post-op chemotherapy (usually FOLFOX) or further chemo if unresectable Can consider short-course pre-op RT rather than chemoRT for select patients |
| Resectable M1, synchronous with primary | Chemo (FOLFOX or FOLFIRI ± bevacizumab or ± panitumumab or cetuximab if KRAS wildtype) → staged or synchronous resection of metastatic lesion(s) and primary rectal tumor, with consideration of pre-op chemoRT before resection of primary |
| Unresectable M1, synchronous with primary | Chemo ± palliative RT ± palliative surgical procedure (diverting ostomy) |

Trans-abdominal excision can consist of low anterior resection (LAR) for mid to upper tumors or abdominoperineal resection (APR) for low tumors, with total mesorectal excision (TME).

## TECHNICAL CONSIDERATIONS

### Simulation
- Simulate prone with belly board and a full bladder to displace small bowel
- PO contrast
- Anal marker or wire perineal scar if present

### Dose Prescription
- Pre-op chemoRT:
  - Pelvis to 45 Gy in 1.8 Gy/fx
  - Sequential tumor boost to 50.4 Gy in 1.8 Gy/fx
- Pre-op RT:
  - 25 Gy in 5 Gy/fx
- Post-op chemo-RT:
  - Pelvis to 45 Gy in 1.8 Gy/fx
  - Sequential tumor bed boost to 50.4 to 54 Gy in 1.8 Gy/fx if negative margins or 54 to 59.4 Gy in 1.8 Gy/fx if positive margins, or
  - Dose painted IMRT with 54 Gy in 2 Gy/fx to tumor bed and 45.9 to 48.6 Gy in 1.7 to 1.8 Gy/fx to pelvic nodes.
- Definitive ChemoRT:
  - Pelvis to 45 Gy in 1.8 Gy/fx, tumor boost to 54 to 59.4 Gy in 1.8 Gy/fx if attainable within normal tissue constraints

### Target Delineation
Contour on soft tissue windows

- GTV = Primary tumor based on exam, endoscopic findings, and imaging. For post-op treatment, fuse pre-op imaging to define tumor bed.
- CTV = GTV (or tumor bed) + 2- to 3-cm margin, perirectal, presacral, and internal iliac nodes. Add external iliac nodes for T4 tumors or extension to the anal canal. Consider adding inguinal nodes if anal canal involved, using intensity-modulated radiation therapy (IMRT) to decrease dose to normal tissues. Add the perineal wound if post-abdominoperineal resection (APR).

■ PTV = CTV + 0.5 to 0.7 cm with daily image-guided radiation therapy.

### Treatment Planning
■ 3D conformal is standard
■ Consider IMRT in select cases (post-op, unable to tolerate prone position, treating inguinal nodes)
■ 6- to 15-MV photons, higher based on patient thickness
■ Pelvis: PA and 2 lateral fields
  ■ PA field borders
    ● Superior—L5/S1
    ● Inferior—3 cm below gross disease, anastomosis (if post-LAR), or including perineal scar (if post-APR)
    ● Lateral—typically 1.5 cm margin on the pelvic brim (adjust according to nodal contours)
  ■ Lateral field borders
    ● Superior and Inferior— same as PA field
    ● Anterior—typically at the posterior margin of pubic symphysis if external iliac nodes not covered or anterior margin of pubic symphysis if covering external iliac nodes (adjust according to nodal contours)
    ● Posterior—behind sacrum
■ Tumor boost: lateral fields, or PA and 2 lateral fields
  ■ Tumor or tumor bed with 2- to 3-cm margin
  ■ Keep posterior border behind the sacrum
■ Heterogeneity corrections used

## FOLLOW UP

If asymptomatic: H&P and carcinoembryonic antigen (CEA) level every 3 to 6 months × 2 years, then every 6 months × 3 years. CT C/A/P every 3 to 6 × 2 years, then every 6 to 12 months × 3 years. Colonoscopy at 1 year and as indicated thereafter.

## SELECTED STUDIES

### Swedish Trial (Folkesson, *J Clin Oncol* 2005; DOI: 10.1200/JCO.2005.08.144)
Patients with stage I to III rectal cancer were randomized to surgery ± neoadjuvant RT consisting of 25 Gy in five fractions over 1 week, delivered within a week of surgery. The addition of neoadjuvant RT improved locoregional recurrence (9% vs. 26%), predominantly for more distal tumors, cancer-specific survival (72% vs. 62%), and overall survival (38% vs. 30%). Surgery was not a total mesorectal excision (TME).

### Dutch Trial (van Gijn, *Lancet Oncol* 2011; DOI: 10.1016/S1470-2045(11)70097-3)

Similar to the Swedish trial, the Dutch trial compared surgery ± neoadjuvant short-course RT to 25 Gy in five fractions. However, surgery consisted of a TME. While neoadjuvant RT reduced local recurrence at 10 years (5% vs. 10%), overall survival was not improved with neoadjuvant RT (48% vs. 49%).

### European Organisation for Research and Treatment of Cancer 22921 (Bosset, *N Engl J Med* 2006; DOI: 10.1056/nejmoa060829)

Four-arm trial comparing neoadjuvant chemoRT ± adjuvant chemotherapy versus neoadjuvant RT ± adjuvant chemotherapy among patients with cT3-4 rectal cancer. RT was 45 Gy in standard fractionation, and surgery included TME for approximately 1/3 of patients. At 5 years, neoadjuvant chemoRT improved locoregional recurrence rates regardless of adjuvant chemotherapy randomization, but did not impact overall survival or disease-free survival (DFS).

### Fédération Francophone de Cancérologie Digestive 9203 (Gérard, *J Clin Oncol* 2006; DOI: 10.1200/JCO.2006.06.7629)

Comparison of neoadjuvant RT (45 Gy in standard fractionation) versus neoadjuvant chemoRT with bolus Fluorouracil (5-FU) and leukovorin, with all patients receiving four cycles of post-op FU/leukovorin. Relative to neoadjuvant RT, neoadjuvant chemoRT improved pathologic complete response rates (11% vs. 4%) and local control (92% vs. 83%), but did not impact rates of sphincter preserving surgery or overall survival.

### German Rectal Cancer Trial (Sauer, *J Clin Oncol* 2012— Long-Term Results; DOI: 10.1200/JCO.2011.40.1836)

Randomized trial comparing neoadjuvant chemoRT to adjuvant chemoRT among patients with T3-4 or node-positive rectal cancer. ChemoRT consisted of 50.4 Gy (additional 5.4 Gy boost for adjuvant arm) along with continuous infusion 5-FU, and adjuvant bolus 5-FU delivered in both arms. Surgery was a TME. Pre-op chemoRT improved locoregional control (7.1% vs. 10.1% at 10 years) and sphincter-preserving surgery in those thought to need an APR, and decreased acute and late treatment-related toxicities, but did not impact progression-free or overall survival (59.6% vs. 59.9% at 10 years).

### Trans Tasman Radiation Oncology Group 01.04 (Ngan, *J Clin Oncol* 2012; DOI: 10.1200/JCO.2012.42.9597)

This trial compared short-course neoadjuvant RT to 25 Gy in five fractions (per Swedish and Danish trials) versus neoadjuvant chemoRT to 50.4 Gy with continuous infusion FU in patients with T3 N0-2 disease. Although there was a higher pathologic complete response in the chemoRT arm, there were no differences in local recurrence rates (7.5% for short-course vs. 4.4% for long-course at 3 years), distant recurrence rates (27% vs. 30% at 5 years), or overall survival (74% vs. 70% at 5 years). For distal tumors, there was a trend toward improved local control with long-course chemoRT.

# 26: ANAL CANCER

*Charles Rutter, MD*
*Kimberly Lauren Johung, MD, PhD*

## WORKUP

### All Cases

- H&P (Rectal and inguinal node exam)
- Anoscopy, possible examination under anesthesia (EUA), and biopsy of primary
- Consider FNA or biopsy of suspicious nodes
- Pelvic exam with pap smear for women
- CT C/A/P ± MRI pelvis with IV contrast
- Consider PET CT for staging and treatment planning
- Consider HIV testing

## TREATMENT RECOMMENDATIONS BY STAGE

| Anal margin (not canal) T1N0 well differentiated | Excise with negative margins |
| --- | --- |
| Localized (any T, any N, M0) | ChemoRT with 5-fluorouracil (FU)/mitomycin or capecitabine/mitomycin |
| Metastatic | Systemic therapy ± palliative RT |
| Local recurrence after chemoRT | Abdominoperineal resection |

## TECHNICAL CONSIDERATIONS

### Simulation

- Supine using custom immobilization or prone with belly board
- PO contrast, consider IV contrast
- Marker at anal verge
- Full bladder for simulation and treatment
- Fuse MRI and PET to sim images

### Dose Prescription

Varies by T & N stage; per RTOG 0529

- For T2N0
    - PTVA (primary tumor): 50.4 Gy in 28 fx of 1.8 Gy
    - PTV42 (nodes): 42 Gy in 28 fx of 1.5 Gy

- For T3-4N0
  - PTVA (primary tumor): 54 Gy in 30 fx of 1.8
  - PTV45 (nodes): 45 Gy in 30 fx of 1.5 Gy
- For N+
  - PTVA (primary tumor): 54 Gy in 30 fx of 1.8 Gy
  - PTV54 (+ LN >3 cm): 54 Gy in 30 fx of 1.8 Gy
  - PTV50 (+ LN ≤3 cm): 50.4 Gy in 30 fx of 1.68 Gy
  - PTV45 (−LN): 45 Gy in 30 fx of 1.5 Gy

**Target Delineation**

Contour using soft tissue windows as per the RTOG anorectal contouring atlas

- GTVA = primary tumor based on exam, CT, MRI, and/or PET
- GTV54 = involved nodes >3 cm
- GTV50 = involved nodes ≤3 cm
- CTVA = GTVA + 2.5 cm, not extending into bone or air
- CTV54: = GTV54 + 1 cm
- CTV50 = GTV50 + 1 cm
- CTV45 or CTV42 = elective nodes
- *7 to 8 mm around iliac vessels, carving out of muscle and bone*
- *Consider 10-mm expansion if nodes identified*
- *Inguinal nodes may be farther from vessels and may need greater expansion*

**CTVA (Perirectal, Presacral, Internal Iliac)**

*Low Pelvis*

- Includes GTVA
- Entire mesorectum to the pelvic floor
- Few mm into levator muscles unless extension into ischiorectal fossa
- 2 cm below gross disease; 2 cm around anal verge
- 1 to 2 cm up to bone around any areas of invasion

*Mid Pelvis*

- Rectum and mesentery
- Internal iliacs with margin for bladder variability
- Posterior and lateral margins to pelvic sidewall musculature or where absent, bone
- Anteriorly, 1 cm into the posterior bladder
- Include at least the posterior internal obturator vessels

*Upper Pelvis*

- Superior extent of perirectal component is the rectosigmoid junction or at least 2 cm proximal to macroscopic disease
- Nodal volume extends up to bifurcation of common iliacs (boney landmark is sacral promontory).

## CTVB (External Iliac)

- Transition from external iliacs to inguinals is at the level of the inferior extent of the internal obturator vessels (boney landmark is upper edge of the superior pubic rami)

## CTVC (Inguinal)

- Contour entire compartment down to 2 cm caudal to the saphenous/femoral junction
- PTV: CTV + 0.5 to 0.7 cm with daily image-guided radiation therapy (IGRT)

## Treatment Planning

- Intensity-modulated radiation therapy
- Usually 6-MV photons
- Use heterogeneity corrections

## FOLLOW UP

Evaluate response at 8 to 12 weeks with digital rectal exam

- If progressive disease, restage
- If locally progressive, salvage abdominoperineal resection (APR)
- If metastatic, systemic therapy (Cisplatin/FU)
- If persistent/stable, re-evaluate in 4 more weeks
- If progressive, manage as noted previously
- If persistent/slowly regressing, continue close monitoring
- Once complete regression achieved:
- H&P, digital rectal exam, and anoscopy q3 to 6 months for 5 years
- CT C/A/P annually for 3 years if T3-4 or N2-3
- Consider surveillance MRIs

## SELECTED STUDIES

### United Kingdom Coordinating Committee on Cancer Research Trial (*Lancet*, 1996; DOI: 10.1016/S0140-6736(96)03409-5)
*ChemoRT versus RT*

First of two randomized trials comparing RT (45 Gy + boost of 15 Gy EBRT or 25 Gy brachytherapy) ± concurrent 5-FU/mitomycin. T1N0 patients were excluded. Local control was significantly improved with chemoRT (61% vs. 39% local control at 3 years), as was anal-cancer specific mortality (28% vs. 39%), although overall survival (OS) was unchanged (65% vs. 58%), likely due to effective salvage surgery.

### EORTC Trial (Bartelink, *J Clin Oncol* 1997; http://jco.ascopubs.org/content/15/5/2040.abstract)
*ChemoRT versus RT*

The second historical trial randomizing patients to RT (45 Gy + 15–20 Gy boost) ± concurrent 5-FU/mitomycin. This trial specifically required patients to be T3-4 and/or N+. ChemoRT improved 5-year locoregional control (68% vs. 50%), colostomy-free survival (72% vs. 40%), and progression-free survival (61% vs. 43%). As in the United Kingdom Coordinating Committee on Cancer Research (UKCCR) study, there was no difference in overall survival (57% vs. 52%) due to effective salvage surgery.

### Intergroup Trial (Flam, *J Clin Oncol* 1996; http://jco.ascopubs.org/content/14/9/2527.abstract)
*Role of Mitomycin*

Because of the significant hematologic toxicity of mitomycin, the Intergroup trial investigated the effectiveness of FU-based chemoRT to 45 to 50.4 Gy ± mitomycin in a cohort of 310 anal cancer patients with any stage of disease. The mitomycin-containing arm had significantly lower colostomy rates (9% vs. 23%), as well as improved colostomy-free survival (71% vs. 59%), and disease-free survival (73% vs. 51%), albeit at the expense of higher grade 4 to 5 toxicity (23% vs. 7%).

### RTOG 9811 (Gunderson, *J Clin Oncol* 2012—Long-term Results; DOI: 10.1200/JCO.2012.43.8085)
*5-FU/Mitomycin versus Induction and Concurrent 5-FU/Cisplatin*

This trial randomized patients with T2-4 N0-3 anal cancer to 5-FU/mitomycin chemoRT to 45 to 59 Gy versus induction chemotherapy (two cycles of 5-FU/cisplatin) followed by 5-FU/cisplatin chemoRT to 45 to 59 Gy. Because this trial essentially addresses two separate questions, including the benefit of induction chemotherapy and the efficacy of cisplatin in place of mitomycin, the results are somewhat difficult to interpret. Nevertheless, 5-year outcomes were improved with 5-FU/mitomycin (disease-free survival 68% vs. 58%; OS 78% vs. 71%; colostomy-free survival 72% vs. 65%).

### ACT-II Trial (James, *Lancet Oncol* 2013; DOI: 10.1016/S1470-2045(13)70086-X)

*5-FU/Mitomycin versus 5-FU/Cisplatin; Maintenance Chemotherapy*

Two questions were addressed by this trial using a $2 \times 2$ randomization. Patients without metastatic disease were randomized to receive chemoRT to 50.4 Gy, with 5-FU/mitomycin versus 5-FU/cisplatin, and to receive two cycles of maintenance 5-FU/cisplatin or undergo observation after chemoRT. At median follow-up of 5 years, there were no significant differences in colonoscopy free survival (CFS), PFS, or OS between patients based upon receipt of mitomycin/FU versus cisplatin/FU, and there was no benefit observed with maintenance chemotherapy after chemoRT.

### RTOG 0529 (Kachnic, *Int J Radiat Oncol Biol Phys* 2013; DOI: 10.1016/j.ijrobp.2012.09.023)

*IMRT*

Phase II trial evaluating dose-painted IMRT for T2-4 N0-3 anal cancer, using target delineation and dose guidelines. When compared to the toxicity profile of conventionally designed radiotherapy (on RTOG 9811), IMRT improved grade 2+ hematologic and grade 3+ dermatologic and GI toxicity, with comparable local control rates.

### Contouring Atlas (Myerson, *Int J Radiat Oncol Biol Phys* 2009; DOI: 10.1016/j.ijrobp.2008.08.070)

Elective clinical target volumes for conformal therapy in anorectal cancer: a radiation therapy oncology group consensus panel contouring

# 27: OVARIAN CANCER

*Jacqueline Kelly, MD, MSc*
*Melissa Young, MD, PhD*
*Shari Damast, MD*

## WORKUP

### All Cases

- H&P (pelvic exam, family history, refer for genetic counseling if indicated)
- Transvaginal ultrasound and/or abdominal/pelvic CT/MRI
- GI evaluation as clinically indicated
- Chest imaging (CXR or CT)
- CBC, BUN/Cr, LFTs, CA-125
- CEA, CA 19-9 as clinically indicated
- Pathologic confirmation: laparotomy, collect ascites/washings, total abdominal hysterectomy bilateral salpingo oophorectomy (TAH/BSO), complete abdominal exploration, omentectomy, random peritoneal biopsies, aortic/pelvic lymph node dissection

### If <40 Years Old

AFP and $\beta$HCG to rule out germ cell tumors. Consultation with reproductive endocrinologist.

## TREATMENT RECOMMENDATIONS BY STAGE

| IA/B Gr 1 | Surgery → observation |
|---|---|
| IA/B Gr 2 | Surgery → observation<br>OR Surgery → taxane/carboplatin × 3–6c |
| IA/B Gr 3, IC, or clear cell | Surgery → taxane/carboplatin × 3–6c |
| II—IV | Surgery → taxane/carboplatin × 6c<br>OR 3–6c of chemo → surgical staging → 3–6c chemo |
| Abdominal/ pelvic recurrence | >6 months from completion of primary therapy: retreat with same agents<br><6 months from completion of primary therapy: consider additional systemic agents; if isolated, consider surgery followed by chemo<br>May consider involved field RT for localized recurrence or palliation |
| WART | Currently not routinely used, but is an option for Stages I–III if not chemo candidate and residual disease <2 cm |

c = cycles; WART = whole abdominal radiation therapy.

## TECHNICAL CONSIDERATIONS

### Simulation
- Patient supine with alpha cradle
- If WART, consider 4D scan to allow customized shielding during respiration

### Dose Prescription
*Involved Field RT for Locoregionally Recurrent*
- Consider standard fractionation to dose of 45 to 60 Gy as appropriate
- May or may not include adjacent nodal basins
- IMRT or 3DCRT + brachytherapy may be appropriate

*For WART*
- 22.5 to 30 Gy in 1.2 to 1.5 Gy/fx to whole field; block kidneys at 18 Gy, block liver at 25 Gy
- Paraaortic boost to 45 Gy
- Pelvis boost to 45 to 50.4 Gy
- May consider IMRT

### Target Delineation
*If Involved Field for Locoregionally Recurrent Disease*
- Primary GTV = gross disease
- Primary clinical target volume (CTV) = post-op bed or prechemo extent of disease + 1- to 1.5- cm margin, exclude uninvolved clinical structures
- *Note*: Patients may have had multiple regional recurrences at the same or nearby regions. Therefore, for CTV delineation, it is important to critically examine *all previous imaging* studies to ensure adequate coverage of regions at risk.
- Nodal CTV—include grossly involved nodes, may extend to cover adjacent uninvolved regions.

*For WART*
Treat AP/PA. Borders: superior = above diaphragm; inferior = below obturator foramen; lateral = beyond peritoneal reflection.

### Treatment Planning
*If involved field for locoregionally recurrent disease*
- IMRT or 3DCRT + brachytherapy

*For WART*
- Open field technique, often at extended SSD
- IMRT (improved coverage and sparing of OARs) or 3DCRT
- 6- to 10-MV photons

## FOLLOW UP

If asymptomatic: Visits every 2 to 4 months for 2 years, then every 6 months for 3 years, then annually after 5 years; Physical exam including pelvic exam; CA-125 or other tumor markers at each visit if initially elevated; Chest/abdominal/pelvic CT, MRI, or PET-CT as clinically indicated.

## SELECTED STUDIES

### Involved Field Radiation Therapy for Locoregionally Recurrent Ovarian Cancer (Brown, *Gynecol Oncol* 2013; DOI: 10.1016/j.ygyno.2013.04.469)

Retrospective analysis of 102 epithelial ovarian cancer patients treated with definitive IFRT directed to localized nodal and extranodal recurrences. Five-year OS and PFS were 40% and 24%, respectively. Thirty-five percent were NED at median of 38 months after IFRT. Eight clear cell patients had higher 5-year OS and PFS (88%–75%). Definitive IFRT can yield excellent local control and protracted DFS in select patients.

### GOG 7602 (Young, *J Clin Oncol* 2003; DOI: 10.1200/JCO.2003.02.154)

229 patients with Stage IA/B Gr3, 1C or II ovarian cancer without macroscopic residual randomized to $^{32}$P versus cyclophosphamide and cisplatin. Chemo arm showed trends for decreased rate of relapse and rate of death. $^{32}$P arm demonstrated inadequate distribution in 7% and small bowel perforation in 3%, leading authors to conclude chemo is preferred therapy.

### Abdominopelvic Radiotherapy in Ovarian Cancer. A 10-Year Experience (Dembo, *Cancer* 1985; DOI: 10.1002/1097-0142(19850501)55:9+<2285:: AID-CNCR2820551436>3.0.CO;2-4)

190 patients with Stage IB, II, asymptomatic III randomized to pelvic RT versus pelvic RT + chlorambucil versus WART. In patients with complete resection, WART improved 5- and 10-year OS versus pelvic RT + chlorambucil (10-year OS 64 vs. 40%).

**High-Risk Early Stage Ovarian Cancer. Randomized Clinical Trial Comparing Cisplatin Plus Cyclophosphamide versus Whole Abdominal Radiotherapy (Chiara, *Am J Clin Oncol* 1994; DOI: 10.1097/00000421-199402000-00016)**

Only randomized trial using modern chemo versus. WART, closed early due to protocol violations and low accrual. 70 patients randomized, 5-year OS 71% for chemo arm and 53% for WART ($p = .16$). Toxicity worse in WART arm.

**Low-Stage Ovarian Clear Cell Carcinoma: Population-Based Outcomes in British Columbia, Canada With Evidence for a Survival Benefit as a Result of Irradiation (Hoskins, *J Clin Oncol* 2012; DOI: 10.1200/JCO.2011.40.1646)**

Retrospective analysis of 241 Stages I to II clear cell ovarian cancer patients comparing chemo + RT (22.5 Gy/10 fx to pelvis then 22.5 Gy/22 fx to whole abdomen) to chemo alone. RT had no discernible survival benefit for patients with stage IA and IC (rupture alone), but in remainder of patients with stage IC and II, RT improved DFS by 20% at 5 years (relative risk 0.5).

# 28: ENDOMETRIAL CANCER

*Brandon R. Mancini, MD*
*Melissa Young, MD, PhD*
*Shari Damast, MD*

## WORKUP

### All Cases

- H&P (include gynecologic history and pelvic exam)
- Endometrial biopsy (or D&C if inadequate)
- Chest imaging
- CBC

### Considerations

- EUA w/ cystoscopy and/or proctoscopy if clinically or radiographically indicated
- CT Abdomen/pelvis w/ PO and IV contrast
- LFTs, CMP, CA-125
- Genetic testing if age <50 and significant family history of endometrial and/or colorectal malignancies

## TREATMENT RECOMMENDATIONS BY FIGO STAGE FOLLOWING TH/BSO + SURGICAL STAGING

### Early Stage

|     | Grade 1 | Grade 2 | Grade 3[b] |
| --- | --- | --- | --- |
| IA | Observation or IVRT[a] | Observation or IVRT[a] | IVRT |
| IB | IVRT | IVRT | WPRT or IVRT[a] |
| II | WPRT or IVRT | WPRT and/or IVRT | WPRT + IVRT boost |

[a]Consider risk factors, including depth of myometrial invasion, LVSI, lower uterine segment involvement, age >60 years, cervical glandular involvement, large tumor size, and extent of lymphadenectomy.
[b]For high-risk histologies, such as serous, clear cell, undifferentiated, and carcinosarcoma, many add chemotherapy.

## ADVANCED STAGE/INOPERABLE/RECURRENT

| IIIA–IVA | Surgery → ChemoRT → Chemo (preferred)<br>OR surgery → chemo → RT → chemo<br>OR surgery → RT → Chemo |
| --- | --- |
| IVB | Tumor debulking → chemotherapy + RT |

*(continued)*

| Incomplete surgical staging | Imaging + surgical restaging and adjuvant treatment as noted previously |
| --- | --- |
| Medically inoperable | Intracavitary brachytherapy (clinical IA, minimal myometrial invasion grade 1–2) EBRT + ICRT (if >IA) |
| Vaginal cuff recurrence when no prior EBRT | EBRT + brachytherapy + chemotherapy |

## TECHNICAL CONSIDERATIONS

### Simulation for EBRT

Simulate and treat supine with custom immobilization for IMRT. Can consider two scans: One full bladder and one empty bladder fused to create ITV. Utilize IV and PO contrast. Vaginal contrast or tampon can be used to delineate vaginal cuff.

### Dose Prescription for EBRT

- Definitive RT: 45 to 50.4 Gy in 1.8 Gy/fx with consideration of boost for gross pelvic lymph nodes to 60 Gy
- Post-op WPRT: 45 to 50.4 Gy in 1.8 Gy/fx

### Dose Prescription for Brachytherapy

- Post-op high dose rate (HDR) IVRT: 3 × 7 Gy/fx, or 4 × 5.5 Gy/fx, or 5 × 4.7 Gy/fx to 0.5-cm depth
- OR 3 × 10.5 Gy/fx, OR 4 × 8.8 Gy/fx, OR 5 × 7.5 Gy/fx to the vaginal surface
- Post-op HDR IVRT after WPRT to 45 Gy: 2 to 3 × 4 to 5 Gy/fx to 0.5-cm depth
- OR 2-3 × 6.0 Gy/fx to the vaginal surface
- HDR ICRT alone for primary inoperable disease stage IA: 4 × 8.5 Gy/fx, or 5 × 7.3 Gy/fx, or 6 × 6.4 Gy/fx, or 7 × 5.7 Gy/fx prescribed to 2 cm from midpoint of intrauterine source (or to CTV per ABS guidelines)
- HDR ICRT for primary inoperable disease > stage IA, following 45-Gy EBRT: 2 × 8.5 Gy/fx, 3 × 6.3Gy/fx, or 4 × 5.2 Gy/fx prescribed to 2 cm from midpoint of intrauterine source (or to CTV per ABS guidelines)
- HDR IVRT after WPRT to 45 Gy for vaginal cuff recurrence: 5 × 4 to 5.5 Gy/fx to 0.5-cm depth, if tumor thickness <0.5 cm; interstitial brachytherapy if tumor thickness ≥0.5 cm

### Target Delineation

- Post-op IMRT:
    - $CTV_{vaginal\ cuff}$ = Vaginal cuff + incorporation of ITV with additional 1- to 2-cm expansion to account for rectal and bladder filling, as well as vaginal motion
    - $CTV_{vessels}$ = Common, external (down to top of femoral heads), obturator, internal iliac LN regions + presacral LN basin with 7-mm expansion carving out bone, muscle, and organ
    - $PTV_{vaginal\ cuff}$ = $CTV_{vaginal\ cuff}$ + 1.0 cm
    - $PTV_{vessels}$ = $CTV_{vessels}$ + 0.7 cm
    - When treating vaginal cuff in post-op setting with HDR IVRT, it is important for vaginal mucosa to be in contact with cylinder.
    - In post-op vaginal cuff HDR IVRT, treat proximal 3 to 5 cm of vagina with consideration of full-length treatment for high-risk histologies.

### Treatment Planning

- IMRT versus 3DCRT: Typically, IMRT for post-op whole pelvis irradiation.
- High-energy photons.
- At least weekly imaging with port films (MV), kV/kV (institutional preference), or CBCT. Consider daily imaging if IMRT.

## FOLLOW UP

If asymptomatic: H&P every 3 to 6 months × 2 years, then every 6 months or annually thereafter. CA-125 (optional), imaging, and vaginal cytology if clinically indicated.

## SELECTED STUDIES

### PORTEC-1 (Nout, *J Clin Oncol* 2011; DOI: 10.1200/JCO.2010.32.4590)

714 patients with stage IB (G2-3) or IC (G1-2), specifically no IC G3, s/p TAH/BSO, no lymphadenectomy. Randomized to post-op EBRT 46 Gy versus observation. Fifteen-year LRR 5.8% versus 15.5% favoring RT. No OS difference. Higher long-term toxicity with RT.

---

(NOTE: FIGO 1988 staging used in all the selected studies listed)

### GOG-99 (Keys, *Gynecol Oncol* 2004;
DOI: 10.1016/j.ygyno.2003.11.048)
448 patients s/p TAH/BSO + selective pelvic and para-aortic lymph node dissection. Stage IB, IC, and IIA (occult disease). Randomized observation versus post-op pelvic EBRT 50.4 Gy. Decreased 2-year cumulative incidence of recurrence with EBRT (3% vs. 12%). No OS difference.

### MRC ASTEC and NCIC CTG EN.5 (Blake, *Lancet* 2009;
DOI: 10.1016/S0140-6736(08)61767-5)
905 stage I–IIA patients w/ intermediate-risk or high-risk features, including stage IA-IB G3, IC G1-3, serous papillary or clear cell type, and IIA. EBRT 40 to 46 Gy daily versus observation. Brachytherapy allowed by institutional preference in both arms. No OS or DSS difference at 5 years.

### PORTEC-2 (Nout, *J Clin Oncol 2009*;
DOI: 10.1200/JCO.2008.20.2424 & *Lancet* 2010;
DOI: 10.1016/S0140-6736(09)62163-2)
427 patients s/p TAH/BSO w/ high-intermediate risk disease w/ age >60 years and stage IC (G1-2) or stage IB (G3) and stage IIA any age (except G3 with >50% myometrial invasion). PLND not done. Randomized to EBRT 46 Gy versus vaginal apex brachytherapy (HDR or LDR). No significant different in 5-year vaginal recurrence, LRR, DM, or OS. Vaginal RT less toxic, especially GI function and QoL.

### GOG 122 (Randall, *J Clin Oncol* 2006;
DOI: 10.1200/JCO.2004.00.7617)
388 patients w/ stage III–IV s/p TAH/BSO + surgical staging (<2-cm residual tumor). Randomized to WART (30 Gy in 20 fx w/ 15 Gy boost) versus doxorubicin + cisplatin q3w × 8 cycles. Stage-adjusted 5-year PFS and OS better in chemotherapy arm.

### RTOG 9708 (Greven, *Gynecol Oncol* 2006;
DOI: 10.1016/j.ygyno.2006.02.007)
Phase II study of 46 patients s/p TAH/BSO w/ G2-3 and either >50% myometrial invasion, cervical stromal invasion, or pelvic-confined extrauterine disease. WPRT 45 Gy w/ cisplatin → IVRT → 4 cycles cisplatin/paclitaxel. Four-year pelvic, regional, and distant recurrences were 2%, 2%, and 19%, respectively. Four-year OS 85% and DFS 81%. Toxicity G3 (16%) and G4 (5%) reasonable.

**NSGO-9501/EORTC-5591 and MaNGO ILIADE-III Pooled Analysis (Hogberg, *Eur J Cancer* 2010;**

**DOI: 10.1016/j.ejca.2010.06.002)**

Pooled analysis of two randomized trials, including 540 patients w/ stage I–III, s/p TAH/BSO (lymphadenectomy optional). Randomized to adjuvant RT versus adjuvant chemoRT. Five-year PFS better in chemoRT arm with trend toward OS benefit.

# 29: CERVICAL CANCER

*Skyler Johnson, MD*
*Shari Damast, MD*
*Melissa Young, MD, PhD*

## WORKUP

### All Cases

- H&P (complete pelvic, bimanual and rectal exam, supraclavicular nodal exam)
- Smoking cessation
- CBC, complete metabolic profile, urinalysis
- Cervical biopsy (four quadrant or conization)
- Chest imaging

### Considerations

- MRI pelvis
- CT chest/abdomen/pelvis or PET/CT
- Exam under anesthesia, cystoscopy/proctoscopy if concern for bladder/bowel invasion
- Ovarian transposition, reproductive endocrinologist consultation
- HIV testing

## TREATMENT RECOMMENDATIONS BY STAGE

### Primary Therapy

| | |
|---|---|
| IA1 (no lymphovascular space invasion [LVSI]) | Extrafascial hysterectomy or Modified radical hysterectomy (RH) → evaluate risk factors that may require adjuvant treatment *If fertility sparing: Conization with negative margins* |
| IA1 (LVSI) and IA2 | Modified RH + pelvic lymph node dissection (PLND) → evaluate risk factors that may require adjuvant treatmeant OR pelvic RT + brachytherapy *If fertility sparing: Cone biopsy or radical trachelectomy + PLND* |
| IB1 and IIA1 | RH + PLND ± para-aortic sampling → evaluate risk factors that may require adjuvant treatment OR pelvic RT + brachytherapy OR chemoRT (pelvic RT + cisplatin) + brachytherapy *If fertility sparing is desired: Radical trachelectomy + PLND may be considered for IB1* |

(continued)

(*continued*)

| IB2–IVA | ChemoRT + brachytherapy |
| IVB | Chemotherapy<br>OR Chemotherapy + RT or other local treatment in select cases |

### Adjuvant Therapy
- Adjuvant RT if two or more intermediate risk factors: LVSI, >4-cm tumor, >1/3 stromal invasion (Sedlis criteria)
- Adjuvant ChemoRT if one or more high-risk factors: positive margins, parametrial invasion, or positive lymph nodes (Peters criteria)

## TECHNICAL CONSIDERATIONS

### Simulation
- Simulate and treat prone on belly board for intact patients where possible. Utilize PO contrast, bladder filling, and vaginal contrast/markers. Consider marking inferior extent of disease where vaginal extension.
- For adjuvant treatment or intact cervix utilizing IMRT, simulate and treat supine in custom immobilization, bladder full, with PO contrast and vaginal contrast. Consider two scans for bladder full and empty to create internal target volume (ITV). Fuse with MRI/PET imaging (if available) to define tumor extent.

### Dose Prescription
*Definitive Chemoradiation*
- Whole pelvic radiation therapy 45 to 50.4 Gy in 1.8 Gy/fx with consideration for parametrial boost for 50.4 to 54 Gy in 1.8 Gy/fx, and consideration of boosts up to 60 Gy for persistent tumor or bulky nodes. If extended field treatment to include para-aortic nodes indicated, 3DCRT or IMRT to 45 Gy in 1.8 Gy/fx to para-aortic chain and consider boosts up to 60 Gy for positive nodes. Dose-painted IMRT has been described with 55 Gy to positive nodes and 45 Gy to pelvis in 25 fractions.
- Brachytherapy: goal cumulative dose by stage; IA ≥75 Gy; IB–IIB ≥80 to 85 Gy; III–IVA ≥85 to 90 Gy. LDR: 40 to 60 cGy/hr to a total of 40 to 45 Gy to point A (over two insertions). HDR: $4 \times 7$ Gy/fx, $4 \times 6.8$ Gy/fx, $5 \times 6$ Gy/fx, $6 \times 5$ Gy/fx, $5 \times 5.5$ Gy/fx, most now prescribe high-risk CTV D90 receive 100% prescription rather than point A-based dosing.

- Organs at risk dose limits (EQD2 for combined external beam radiation therapy [EBRT] and brachy):
  D2cc bladder <80 to 90 Gy; D2cc sigmoid <70 to 75 Gy; D2cc rectum <70 to 75 Gy, consider D2cc small bowel <60 Gy; vaginal surface max point dose <130 to 140 Gy.

*Adjuvant RT*
WPRT to 45 to 50.4 Gy in 1.8 Gy/fx

## Target Delineation
*External Beam Radiotherapy*
- Pelvic field, four field: superior—L3/L4 or L4/L5; inferior—3 cm below lowest extent or bottom obtu- rator foramen; lateral—2-cm lateral to pelvic brim; anterior—1-cm anterior to pubic symphysis; posterior—at least anterior half of sacrum. Include para-aortic or inguinal as indicated. *Note:* While "classic" pelvic field can be set, goal is to target all suspected disease with 1.5- to 2-cm margin on vessels and 2- to 3-cm margin on vagina/cervix/uterus structures, thus fields should be evaluated to ensure adequate coverage of the nodal and GYN targets described in the following.
  - Nodal targets—common iliacs, external iliac, internal iliac, and obturator nodes and presacral nodal levels. Include para-aortics (if positive or at risk) or inguinals (if lower one-third vaginal involvement).
  - GYN targets—contour uterus, cervix, and any clinical markers or radiographic extent of disease, parametrium, upper half vagina (if no vaginal involvement) or upper two-third vagina (if upper vaginal involvement), or entire vagina (if extensive vaginal involvement). Upper 3 cm of vagina if post-op + any clips.
- Parametrial boosts may be used with midline block to match LDR/HDR treatment, and lowering superior border to exclude small bowel. Conformal nodal boosts may be 3DCRT or IMRT planned with 1- to 1.5-cm margin.

*Brachy*
- For volume-based contouring/dosing, follow GEC-ESTRO guidelines for CT- or MRI-based delineation of CTV$_{High-risk}$. MR based—entire cevix + any parametrial or vaginal extension (gray zones). CT based—all central tissue at level of ring or ovoids, superiorly to internal os, then 1 cm "cone"

along tandem above cervix; laterally, include any parametrial extension (gray/white) or clinical vaginal involvement.

■ For point-based dosing, follow ICRU 38 and 2011 ABS point definitions. Point A—from the intersection of the tandem with a line connecting the top of the ovoids or ring, extends 2-cm above and 2-cm lateral to the tandem (point B 5 cm lateral to tandem). Bladder point—posterior point of midfoley balloon filled with 7-cc fluid. Rectal point—5-mm posterior to vaginal wall at lower intrauterine source. Vaginal surface— surface of ovoids/cylinder.

### Treatment Planning

■ 3DCRT or IMRT: Typically IMRT for post-op whole pelvis irradiation or extended field RT.

■ High-energy photons.

■ At least weekly imaging with port films (MV), kV/ kV (institutional preference), or cone-beam computed tomography. Consider daily imaging if IMRT.

■ *All RT treatment should be completed in <8 weeks.*

### FOLLOW UP

Consider posttreatment PET after 3 to 4 months. Additional imaging as needed. If asymptomatic, H&P every 3 to 6 months for 2 years, then every 6 to 12 months for 3 to 5 years, then annually thereafter. Cervical cytology with frequency determined by institution.

### SELECTED STUDIES

#### Milan Trial (Landoni, *Lancet* 1997; DOI: 10.1016/S0140-6736(97)02250-2)

337 patients w/FIGO IB-IIA cervical ca randomized to radical hysterectomy and pelvic lymph node dissection versus RT alone. Fifty-four percent in surgery group received adjuvant RT. No diff in overall survival (OS) and disease-free survival (DFS). Worse toxicity in surgery arm.

#### GOG 92 (Sedlis, *Gynecol Oncol* 1999; DOI: 10.1006/gyno.1999.5387)

277 patients w/FIGO IB cervical ca s/p radical hysterectomy and pelvic lymph node dissection with two risk factors: LVSI, >1/3 stromal invasion or tumor size ≥4 cm, randomized to adjuvant WPRT versus observation. +LN excluded. RT improved progression-free survival.

### GOG 109 (Peters, *J Clin Oncol* 2000; http://jco.ascopubs.org/content/18/8/1606.long)

243 patients w/FIGO IA$_2$-IIA cervical ca s/p hysterectomy and pelvic lymph node dissection with high-risk feature(s): +LN, +margin, +parametria randomized to adjuvant WPRT versus adjuvant WPRT and cisplatin/5-FU. CRT improved PFS (80% vs. 63%) and OS (81% vs. 71%) versus RT alone.

### RTOG 9001 (Morris, *N Engl J Med* 1999; DOI: 10.1056/NEJM199904153401502 and Eiffel, *J Clin Oncol* 2004; DOI: 10.1200/JCO.2004.07.197)

389 patients w/FIGO IIB-IVA or IB-IIA tumor >5 cm or +LN (excluded patients with + para-aortic LN) cervical ca randomized to WPRT with concurrent cisplatin/5-FU + brachy versus extended field RT + brachy. Improved DFS (67% vs. 40%) and OS (73% vs. 58%) with chemoRT. Acute toxicity worse (11% vs. 1%) with chemoRT, no difference in late toxicity.

### GOG 120 (Whitney, *J Clin Oncol* 1999; http://jco.ascopubs.org/content/17/5/1339.full.pdf and Rose, *J Clin Oncol* 2007; DOI: 10.1200/JCO.2006.09.4532)

526 patients w/IIB-IVA randomized to cisplatin, cisplatin/5-FU/hydroxyurea, or hydroxyurea. All received pelvic RT + brachy. Platinum-based chemotherapy improves PFS (46%/43%/26%) and OS (53%/53%/34%).

### Argentinian (Duenas-Gonzalez, *J Clin Oncol* 2011; DOI: 10.1200/JCO.2009.25.9663)

515 patients w/FIGO IIB-IVA cervical ca randomized to WPRT + gem/cis followed by brachy then two cycles gem/cis versus WPRT + cisplatin followed by brachy. Gem/cis arm improved PFS and OS but more toxic.

# 30: VAGINAL CANCER

*Debra Nana Yeboa, MD*
*Shari Damast, MD*
*Melissa Young, MD, PhD*

## WORKUP

### All Cases

- H&P (include sexual partners, smoking history, Gyn and anorectal symptoms)
- Gyn exam, pap smear, colposcopy, vulvar evaluation
- Rule out synchronous anorectal, cervical or vulvar primary with vaginal metastasis or extension
- EUA with biopsies (consider cystoscopy/proctoscopy)

### Considerations

- HPV and HIV status
- MRI pelvis with vaginal contrast and/or vaginal cylinder and IV contrast
- PET or CT abdomen/pelvis, CXR

## TREATMENT RECOMMENDATIONS BY STAGE

| | |
|---|---|
| I<br>≤0.5-cm thick | [a]RT is preferred in most cases for organ preservation<br>EBRT + brachytherapy<br>OR brachytherapy alone (only in select favorable cases or vaginal intra-epithelial neoplasia)<br>*Surgery*<br>• upper vagina, radical vaginectomy, and pelvic LND with neovagina reconstruction<br>• lower third vagina, include inguinal LND<br>• option for total vaginectomy for squamous cell carcinoma only; with adenocarcinoma radical vaginectomy for concern of subepithelial spread |
| I<br>>0.5-cm thick | *RT*<br>• EBRT + brachytherapy<br>*Surgery*<br>• upper vagina, radical vaginectomy, and pelvic LND with neovagina construction<br>• lower third vagina, include inguinal LND |
| II | EBRT + brachytherapy<br>consider concurrent chemotherapy[b] |

*(continued)*

| III | ChemoRT[b] + brachytherapy[a] |
|-----|-------------------------------|
| IVA | ChemoRT[b] + brachytherapy[a] |
| IVB | RT for palliation + chemotherapy |

[a]EBRT boost may be considered in select cases, *i.e.*, distal vagina/rectovaginal septum/bladder involvement.
[b]Concurrent chemotherapy has been shown in many series to improve outcomes and is often used in stage II–IV disease.

## TECHNICAL CONSIDERATIONS

### Simulation

- Simulate supine, frog-legged with custom immobilization, full bladder, PO contrast. Consider bladder full and empty scans to generate vaginal ITV. Consider IV contrast.
- Place markers at tumor for delineation and fuse with MRI/ PET imaging (if available) to define tumor extent

### Dose Prescription

*Initial Fields*
EBRT pelvis (+ inguinal nodes if lower vagina involved) 45 Gy in 1.8 Gy/fx (+ pelvic side wall/nodal boosts to 54–66 Gy in 1.8–2 Gy/fx)

*Boost to Primary Disease*
Brachytherapy to 70 to 80 Gy total

- Intracavitary (<5-mm gross disease thickness)
- May be done with single channel, multichannel, or partially shielded vaginal cylinder applicators
- Interstitial (>5-mm gross disease thickness)—Syed applicator; consider referral to treatment center with specialist/expertise

Common HDR fractionation = $5 \times 4.5 - 5.5$ Gy/fx after EBRT 45 Gy to pelvis
   Other considerations:

- If bulky tumor and/or poor response to EBRT, may consider brachytherapy dose escalation up to 85 Gy total dose; some treat entire vagina to 60 Gy cumulative, followed by tumor boost to 75 to 85 Gy
   If not a candidate for brachytherapy, may consider boost with IMRT to 75 Gy

## Target Delineation

### EBRT

- $GTV_{primary}$ = Primary tumor delineated by exam, EUA op note, diagrams, and fusion with MRI pelvis and/or PET/CT.
- $CTV_{primary}$ = Entire vagina, paravaginal tissues, and GTV with 1- to 2-cm margin. Account for possible internal organ motion as vaginal apex can move up to 2 cm in AP direction.
- $CTV_{pelvis/nodes}$ = Pelvic nodal coverage of common iliac, internal and external iliac, presacral, and obturator nodes, and if lower third vaginal lesion include inguinal nodes. Contour vessels with 7-mm brush editing bone/muscle/bowel, but note that inguinal nodes can lie up to 2 to 3 cm from vessels, so contour based on patient anatomy.
- PTV = Per institutional required margin to account for set-up error based on image verification available, often 0.7 to 1 cm.
- Inferior field border should extend approximately 3 cm below the inferior extent of vaginal disease.

### Brachytherapy

Brachytherapy planning is highly individualized and should incorporate information from pre-EBRT and pre-brachytherapy imaging (preferably MRI), fiducials, and exam findings. Careful understanding of vaginal anatomy and distribution of disease is required. 3D-based planning strongly encouraged. Tumor extent, location, and response must all be considered when choosing brachytherapy approach.

## Treatment Planning

### EBRT

- 3DCRT or IMRT
- High energy photons
- Minimum weekly ports; daily IGRT especially if IMRT utilized.

### Brachytherapy

- 3D image-guided planning encouraged
- Attention to vaginal surface dose and surrounding dose to OARs
- Use EQD2 dose conversions (available as spreadsheet on ABS website) to track dose to normal tissues

## FOLLOW UP

If asymptomatic: First 2 years q3 months, next 3 years q 6 months, then annually. Cytology and imaging as indicated.

## SELECTED STUDIES

### Frank et al. (*Int J Radiat Oncol Biol Phys* 2005; DOI: 10.1016/j.ijrobp.2004.09.032)

Retrospective review from MDACC from 1970 to 2000, 193 patients, invasive SCC only, treated with definitive RT [stage I (26%), stage II (50%), stage III (20%), stage IVA (4%)], among stage III to IV, 5% received neoadjuvant chemo and 17% received concurrent ChemoRT. Five-year pelvic control stage I (86%), II (84%), III to IVA (71%), worse for patients with >4-cm tumors (85% ≤4 cm vs. 75% >4cm). Five-year DSS stage I (85%), II (78%), III to IVA (58%). Five-year DSS ≤4-cm tumor 82% vs. >4 cm 60%. Predominate mode of relapse was local-regional (stage I–II 68% vs. stage III–IV 83%).

### Creasman et al. (*Cancer* 1998; DOI: 10.1002/(SICI) 1097-0142(19980901)83:5<1033::AID-CNCR30>3.0.CO;2-6)

National cancer database report of vaginal cancers, 1985 to 1994 of 4,885 cases, several histologies. Relative survival at 5 years: stage 0 (in situ) 96%, stage I (73%), stage II (58%), stage III to IV (36%).

### Rajagopalan et al. (*Gynecol Oncol* 2014; DOI: 10.1016/j.ygyno.2014.09.018)

National cancer database report, 1998 to 2011, comparison of patients of all stages (I, II, III, IV) receiving RT alone versus chemotherapy and RT. Median survival by stage I (RT alone, 83 vs. CRT, 109 months); II (RT alone, 42 vs. CRT, 86 months); III (RT alone, 20 vs. CRT, 43 months); IV (RT alone, 9 vs. CRT, 19 months).

### Kim et al. (*Pract Radiat Oncol* 2012; DOI: 10.1016/j.prro.2011.12.005)

Imaging from 22 patients with pelvic malignancies and positive inguinal nodes were reviewed, measuring distance of positive node to femoral vessel. Distance of nodal areas from femoral vessels were >2 cm in most directions. Exercise caution in extrapolating pelvic nodal contouring guidelines to inguinal lymph nodal contouring. Contouring LN as a compartment defined by anatomic landmarks may be more reproducible.

# 31: VULVAR CANCER

*Trevor Bledsoe, MD*
*Shari Damast, MD*
*Melissa Young, MD, PhD*

## WORKUP

### All Cases
- H&P
- Smoking cessation assistance if indicated
- Labs—CBC, CMP, UA
- PAP smear, digital rectal exam

### Considerations
- HPV testing
- Examination under anesthesia: cystoscopy or proctoscopy as indicated
- Imaging: CT abdomen/pelvis or PET/CT. Consider MRI for advanced disease

## TREATMENT RECOMMENDATIONS BY STAGE

| | |
|---|---|
| Early stage T1, small T2 without involvement of anus, vagina, or urethra | Surgical resection<br>• Wide local excision for ≤1-mm invasion<br>• Radical local resection or modified radical vulvectomy if >1-mm invasion with nodal evaluation<br>  • Bilateral nodal eval for midline lesions<br>  • Unilateral nodal eval for lesions ≥2 cm from vulvar midline (can consider sentinel lymph node [SLN] if not multi-focal)<br>• Re-excision for positive margin if resectable<br>Adjuvant radiation therapy to vulva considered for:<br>• Unresectable positive margins<br>• Close margins (<8 mm)<br>• Tumor >4 cm<br>• Extensive lymphovascular space invasion (LVSI) or deeply invasive disease<br>Adjuvant RT or ChemoRT to inguinal/pelvic nodes if >1 LN+ or LN metastasis >2 mm or ECE on SLN or nodal dissection, gross residual disease |

*(continued)*

*(continued)*

| Locally advanced<br>• Large T2, T3<br>• surgery would be nonorgan preserving<br>• Fixed/ulcerated LN | Primary or neoadjuvant ChemoRT for unresectable disease (± upfront surgical nodal evaluation)<br>• If CR—consider biopsy and if negative—observe<br>• If no response/partial response, resection if feasible, if not resectable, individualized RT ± chemo or supportive care |
|---|---|
| Distant metastatic<br>(Stage IVB) | Chemotherapy<br>RT for locoregional control and/or palliation |

*CRT—concurrent chemoradiotherapy; usually cisplatin containing*

### TECHNICAL CONSIDERATIONS

#### Simulation

Simulate and treat with patient supine, frog-legged with custom immobilization with full bladder. Oral contrast. Place radiopaque markers on surgical incision sites, palpable nodes, gross disease, and anal verge. Consider bolus on incision sites and perineum. Fuse MRI if available.

#### Dose Prescription

*Pre-Op*

- 45 to 60 Gy in 1.8 Gy/fx to primary ± groins/pelvis depending on LN risk

*Definitive ChemoRT*

- 45 Gy in 1.8 Gy/fx to primary/vulva/pelvis/groins followed by cone-down to total of 60 to 65 Gy to gross primary and nodal disease.

*Adjuvant RT*

- 45 to 50.4 Gy in 1.8 Gy/fx. If for positive margin and/or gross residual up to 60 to 65 Gy in 1.8 Gy/fx

#### Target Delineation

*Definitive/Pre-Op*

- GTV = all gross disease and involved/suspicious enlarged lymph nodes on physical exam, imaging, etc.
- CTV = GTV + 1 to 2 cm and should include the entire vulva, inguinal-femoral nodes, and pelvic lymph nodes. Inguinal nodal CTV may be up to 2 to 3 cm around vessels
- Inferior field border should extend at least 2 cm below vulvar disease extent

*Boost*
- GTV: all gross disease (primary tumor, involved nodes)
- CTV: GTV + 1 to 2 cm

*Adjuvant*
- CTV is vulva ± pelvic and inguinal nodes.

**Treatment Planning**
- 3DCRT or IMRT; Multiple 3D techniques for pelvic field plus inguinal coverage to allow for dose sparing of the femoral neck: "photon thunderbird," "modified segmental boost technique," electron tags. Less long-term data for IMRT.
- Add bolus to ensure adequate dose to the vulva target volume
- In vivo dosimetry to ensure adequate skin coverage
- Photons ± electrons depending on treatment methods for groins. If using AP/PA treatment portals, 6 MV used for the anterior field with high energy beams posteriorly.
- Consider daily image-guided radiation therapy, especially if IMRT

**FOLLOW UP**

H&P every 3 to 6 months for 2 years, then every 6 to 12 months for 3 to 5 years. Follow-up imaging based on symptoms or atypical exam findings. Cervical/vaginal cytology as indicated

**SELECTED STUDIES**

**GOG 36 (Homesley HD, *Gynecol Oncol* 1993;
DOI: 10.1006/gyno.1993.1127)**
Prospective staging trial; 588 patients with squamous cell carcinoma (SCC) of the vulva treated from 1977 to 1984. Statistically significant independent predictors of positive groin nodes were (in order of importance): higher grade, suspicious or fixed/ulcerated lymph nodes, presence of capillary–lymphatic involvement, older age, and greater tumor thickness.

**GOG 37 (Kunos, *Obstet Gynecol* 2009;
DOI: 10.1097/AOG.0b013e3181b12f99)**
114 patients with SCC of the vulva underwent radical vulvectomy and bilateral inguinal lymph node dissection (LND), if positive nodes, randomized to ipsilateral pelvic LN dissection or RT to bilateral groin and pelvic nodes. No RT delivered to vulva primary lesion. RT arm with superior CSS at 6 years (71% vs. 49%) and

overall survival among those with cN2-N3 disease or ≥ 2 positive LNs. Ratio of ≥20% positive ipsilateral LNs was associated with contralateral LN metastasis, relapse, and cancer-related death.

### Heaps (Gynecol Oncol 1990; DOI: 10.1016/0090-8258(90)90064-R)

Review of 135 patients with SCC of the vulva to identify surgical-pathologic variables predictive of local recurrence. Surgical margin <8 mm most powerful predictor of local recurrence. Other significant factors included: depth of invasion, increasing tumor thickness, infiltrative growth, LVSI, increasing keratin, and >10 mitoses per 10 hpf.

### GOG 88 (Stehman, Int J Radiat Oncol Biol Phys 1992; DOI: 10.1016/0360-3016(92)90699-I)

Planned for 300 patients T1-T3, nonsuspicious inguinal nodes, randomized to bilateral inguinal/femoral LND versus bilateral groin RT (50 Gy to 3 cm depth). Prematurely stopped at 52 patients due to 18% of RT patients and 0% LND patients with recurrence. OS RT 63% versus 88% surgery. Criticisms include 3-cm prescription depth underdosed nodes in most patients.

### GOG 101 (Moore, Int J Radiat Oncol Biol Phys 1998; DOI: 10.1016/S0360-3016(98)00193-X)

Phase II study; 73 patients with T3-T4 SCC of the vulva who underwent planned split course RT with concurrent cisplatin/Fluorouracil (5-FU) followed by resection of primary and bilateral inguinal-femoral LND. RT dose was 4760 cGy; 170 cGy/fx delivered twice a day (BID), days 1 to 4 of each course and qd days 5 to 12. Two-week break between courses of RT. Complete response in 47%; 2.8% of patients had residual, unresectable disease. Survival rate of 55% at 50 months.

### GOG 205 (Moore, Gynecol Oncol 2012; DOI: 10.1016/j.ygyno.2011.11.003)

Phase II study of 58 patients that evaluated RT (57.6 Gy/1.8 Gy per fraction) with concurrent, weekly cisplatin (40 mg/m$^2$) for patients with locally advanced, unresectable vulvar carcinoma. 69% of patients completed treatment. Complete clinical response was seen in 37 patients (64%). Complete pathological response in 78% of patients who underwent biopsy. RT + weekly cisplatin yielded high rates of complete clinical and pathologic response with acceptable toxicity.

**(GROINSS-V)I (Te Grootenhuis, *J Clin Oncol* 2008; *Gynecol Oncol* 2016; DOI: 10.1097/AOG.0b013e3181b12f99)**

403 patients, prospective trial that included patients with T1-2 <4 cm squamous cell carcinoma of the vulva and clinically negative inguinal nodes. SLN performed and if negative LND omitted. At 3 years, 2.3% groin failure in SLN-negative patients, with OS of 97%. Lymphedema rate (2% vs. 25%) and recurrent erysipelas (0.4% vs. 16%) less in SLN-negative patients versus LND. 10-year results in 377 patients with unifocal disease found DSS 91% for SLN-negative patients compared to 65% for SLN-positive patients (*P* <.0001) and low rates of isolated groin failure, but local recurrence rates high in both groups 36% versus 46.4%.

# 32: PROSTATE INTACT

*Gary Walker, MD*
*Deborah A. Kuban, MD*

## WORKUP

### All Cases

- H&P (comorbidities/life expectancy, urinary and erectile function, digital rectal exam)
- PSA (doubling time, density)
- Transrectal ultrasound guided biopsy
- Gleason Score (GS)

### Considerations

- Bone scan if T1 and PSA >20, T2 and PSA >10, GS ≥8, T3/4 or symptomatic
- Pelvic CT or MRI if T1/2 and nomogram probability of lymph nodes >10%, or T3/T4
- Evaluate for pubic arch interference if considering brachytherapy.

## TREATMENT RECOMMENDATIONS BY STAGE

| | | |
|---|---|---|
| Very low risk: T1c, ≤GS6, ≤PSA 10, <3 cores, ≤50% cancer in each core, PSA density <0.15 ng/mL/g | LE ≥20 years | Active surveillance OR EBRT, OR brachytherapy, OR radical prostatectomy (RP) OR SBRT (ideally on trial) |
| | LE 10 to 20 years | Active surveillance |
| | LE <10 years | Observation |
| Low risk: ≤T2a, ≤GS6, ≤PSA 10 | LE ≥10 years | Active surveillance, OR EBRT, OR brachytherapy, OR RP OR SBRT (ideally on trial) |
| | LE <10 years | Observation |
| Intermediate risk: T2b-T2c, or GS7, or PSA 10.1 to 20 | RP + pelvic lymph node dissection (PLND) | |
| | EBRT + androgen deprivation therapy (ADT) (4–6 months) ± brachy OR brachy alone | |
| | Consider observation (if LE <10 years) | |

*(continued)*

(*continued*)

| High risk:<br>T3, or GS ≥8, or<br>PSA ≥20 | EBRT + ADT (2–3 years)<br>OR EBRT + Brachy ± ADT (2–3 years) |
|---|---|
| | RP + PLND |

## TECHNICAL CONSIDERATIONS

### Simulation

- Enema 1 hour prior to minimize prostate distortion by full rectum.
- Full Bladder. Have patient drink (18–24 oz water 30–60 minutes prior) to push bowel away
- Rectal balloon (if needed) to immobilize prostate and push sigmoid away
- MedTech™ or Vac-Lok™ to immobilize lower extremities.
- Isocenter in the mid-plane mid-prostate.

### Dose Prescription

- Definitive RT:
  - 75.6 to 81 Gy in 1.8 to 2 Gy/fx.

- Hypofractionated radiation therapy:
  - 2.4 to 4 Gy/fx over 4 to 6 weeks (several regimens reported with varying follow-up and acceptable toxicity).

- SBRT:
  - 7.25 to 8 Gy/fx × 5 fx with varying follow-up and toxicity

- Brachytherapy:
  - 145 Gy to the PTV for Iodine 125, 125 Gy to the PTV for Pd-103, and 115 Gy to the PTV for Cs-131.

### Target Delineation

*EBRT:*

Contour prostate and seminal vesicles (SV)

- CTV =
  - Low risk—prostate (+proximal SV if large tumor burden at base), intermediate risk—prostate + proximal SV, high risk—Prostate + full SV (if normal tissue tolerance allows).
  - PTV = 6-mm expansion except 4 mm posteriorly.

- Brachytherapy:
  - PTV—3 mm radially except 0 mm posteriorly, 5 mm superior/inferior
- SBRT:
  - PTV 3- to 5-mm margins (reduced to 3 mm or less posteriorly), or per trial protocol
  - Consider pelvic lymph node radiation for high-risk disease.
  - Daily prostate localization should be used (implanted fiducials with daily kV imaging, daily CT, or electromagnetic targeting)

**Treatment Planning**
- Highly conformal techniques should be used, preferably IMRT.
- Volumetric arc therapy reduces treatment time and may provide better conformality
- 6-MV photons instead of 18 MV to reduce neutron component
- Rectum V70 Gy <20%, V75 Gy <15%. Bladder V70 Gy <20%.

**FOLLOW UP**

PSA q6 to12 months for 5 years
DRE yearly (may be omitted if PSA undetectable)

**SELECTED STUDIES**

**Klotz Active Surveillance (Klotz, *J Clin Oncol* 2014; DOI: 10.1200/JCO.2014.55.1192)**
450 patients with mostly low-risk disease underwent PSA q3mo × 2 years then q6 months and repeat biopsy at 6 to12 months and q3 to 4 years until age 80. Treated if PSA doubling time <3 years, progression to GS7 or nodule. Patients remaining on surveillance: 5 years = 76%, 10 years = 64%, 15 years = 55%. Excellent cause specific survival (CSS) (94.3% at 15 years).

**MD Anderson Dose Escalation (Kuban, *Int J Radiat Oncol Biol Phys* 2008; DOI: 10.1016/j.ijrobp.2007.06.054)**
301 T1-T3 patients, stratified by PSA <10 (65%), 10 to 20 (35%), >20 (few) randomized to 70 Gy versus 78 Gy. No ADT. Dose escalation improved 8-year PSA FFF (78% vs. 59% SS). No overall survival (OS) difference. GI Grade 3 toxicity was higher with

dose escalation, 7% versus 1% SS, but study was prior to the use of dose-volume histogram (DVH) criteria.

### RTOG 94-08 (Jones, *N Engl J Med* 2011; DOI: 10.1056/NEJMoa1012348)

1979 men with T1b-2b, PSA <20, any GS received whole pelvis (66.6 Gy) or prostate only (68.4 Gy) depending on risk factors. Randomized ± 2 months neoadjuvant and 2 months concurrent ADT. ADT improved OS (62% vs. 57% SS), reduced biochemical failure (26% vs. 41%). In subset analysis, ADT only supported in intermediate risk and not low risk patients.

### D'Amico Short Course ADT (D'Amico, *JAMA* 2008; DOI: 10.1001/jama.299.3.289)

206 men with intermediate/high risk (T1b-T2b, PSA ≥10, GS ≥7, extracapsular extension (ECE) or T3 on imaging) received 70 Gy prostate only RT. Patients randomized to 6 months ADT beginning 2 months prior to RT. ADT improved 8year OS (74% vs. 61% SS). On subset analysis, benefit was limited to those with none or minimal comorbidities.

### Radiation Therapy Oncology Group 92-02 (Horwitz, *J Clin Oncol* 2008; DOI: 10.1200/JCO.2007.14.9021)

1554 patients with T2c-T4, PSA <150, no common iliac or higher nodes. All patients got ADT 2 months prior to and 2 months during RT (45 Gy whole pelvis + 20–25 Gy boost). Randomized ± 2 years ADT. Long-term ADT reduced PSA failure, local recurrence, distant metastasis, and improved disease-free survival (DFS) and CSS, but OS was improved only in the GS 8 to 10 subgroup.

### European Organisation for Research and Treatment of Cancer 22863 (Bolla, *Lancet Oncol* 2010; DOI: 10.1016/S1470-2045(10)70223-0)

415 patients with T1-2 G3 or T3-4 any grade, N0-1 randomized to RT (50 Gy whole pelvis + 20 Gy prostate boost) versus same RT + 3 year concurrent/adjuvant Goserelin. ADT improved 10-year OS (58% vs. 40% SS). Cancer mortality was reduced from 30% to 10%, and local/regional failure from 24% to 6%. There was no difference in the 10-year incidence of cardiovascular mortality.

# 33: ADJUVANT/SALVAGE PROSTATE CANCER

*Rachit Kumar, MD*
*Deborah A. Kuban, MD*

## WORKUP

### All Cases

- H&P, (life expectancy, comorbidities)
- If salvage, endorectal MRI, CT abdomen/pelvis, bone scan, Prostate-specific antigen (PSA) history, doubling time
- Liver function tests including alkaline phosphatase

### Considerations

- Consider biopsy if prostate bed recurrence seen on imaging or enlarged pelvic nodes

## TREATMENT RECOMMENDATIONS BY STAGE

| pT2N0, + margin | Adjuvant RT to prostate/SV bed |
|---|---|
| pT3/T4 N0 | Adjuvant RT to prostate/SV bed |
| pT3-4 or + margin in pt with N1 disease | Androgen deprivation therapy (ADT) ± RT to prostate bed and nodes |
| Rising PSA s/p radical retropubic prostatectomy (RRP) | Salvage RT to prostate/SV bed. Add nodes if N1. Add ADT for PSA >0.5 to 1.0 ng/mL or other high risk features |

## TECHNICAL CONSIDERATIONS

### Simulation

Simulate with full bladder and empty rectum. Rectal balloon to displace sigmoid colon and small bowel as necessary.

### Dose Prescription

- Adjuvant RT:
  - 64 to 66 Gy in 1.8 to 2.0 Gy/fx
- Salvage RT (No clinical disease in fossa by exam or MRI):
  - 70 Gy in 1.8 to 2.0 Gy/fx
- Salvage RT (Clinical disease in fossa on imaging or exam):
  - 72 to 74 Gy in 1.8 to 2.0 Gy/fx. Entire prostate fossa may be treated to 70 Gy with a boost to the clinical disease to 72 to 74 Gy. Patient should be made aware of the risk of complications with the higher dose levels.

### Target Delineation
### Prostate and SV Bed

Contour using Radiation Therapy Oncology Group (RTOG) atlas for adjuvant/salvage prostate cancer (https://www.rtog.org/CoreLab/ContouringAtlases/ProstatePostOp.aspx).

- Superior—5 mm above the inferior border of the vas deferens remnant.
- Inferior—Top of penile bulb OR 1.5 cm below the urethral beak OR 8 mm below vesicourethral anastomosis
- Anterior—Pubic symphysis at inferior portion, superior to pubic symphysis contour 1 to 2 cm of posterior bladder
- Posterior—Anterior rectum and mesorectal fascia
- Lateral—Medial edge of obturator internus muscle
- Planning target volume (PTV)—5 to 7 mm in all directions, especially 5 mm posteriorly, if daily imaging available. If no daily imaging, use up to 1.0-cm PTV.

### Treatment Planning

- Intensity-modulated radiation therapy (IMRT) strongly recommended to minimize rectal and bladder dose 6 MV for IMRT
- Rectum dose—V70 <20%
- Bladder dose—V50 <50%
- Max sigmoid dose—60 Gy
- Max small bowel dose—50 Gy

Recommend daily bladder US or cone beam computed tomography (CBCT) to confirm bladder filling.

### FOLLOW UP

- H+P and PSA every 3 months × 2 years, then every 6 months years 2 to 5, then annually.
- Imaging only if clinically indicated.

### SELECTED STUDIES

#### SWOG 8794 (Thompson, *J Urology* 2009; DOI: 10.1016/j.juro.2008.11.032)

431 patients with pN0M0 status post-RP with extracapsular extension (ECE), positive margins, or seminal vesicle invasion (SVI). Randomized to RT versus observation (though approx. 1/3 in the obs arm eventually received RT). At 10 years, RT improved overall survival (OS) (74% vs. 66%) and distant metastasis–free survival (DMFS) (71% vs. 61%); and

reduced biochemical failure (47% vs. 74%) and local failure (8% vs. 22%).

### German ARO 96-02 (Wiegel, *Eur Urology* 2014; DOI: 10.1016/j.eururo.2014.03.011)

388 patients with pT3N0 or positive margins s/p radical prostatectomy (RP) randomized to RT versus observation. RT increased progression-free survival (PFS) 56 % versus 35%. Underpowered to assess OS and DMFS

### European Organisation for Research and Treatment of Cancer 22911 (Bolla, *Lancet* 2012; DOI: 10.1016/S0140-6736(12)61253-7)

1005 patients with cT0-3 with pN0 and ECE, pos margins, or SVI s/p RP randomized to RT versus observation (1/2 in obs arm received RT). RT decreased biochemical failure (39% vs. 59%%). No difference in OS and DMFS. Margin status was strongest predictor of benefit.

### Multi-Institutional Salvage RT (Stephenson, *J Clin Oncol* 2007; DOI: 10.1200/JCO.2006.08.9607)

1540 patients with PSA $\geq 0.2$ ng/mL followed by higher value, or single value $\geq 0.5$ ng/mL, all treated with RT, median 64 Gy. Overall 6-year bPFS was 32%. Better outcomes with salvage RT if PSA $\leq 0.2$ ng/mL, Gleason 4 to 7, Positive surgical margins, and PSA doubling time >10 months.

### Johns Hopkins Retrospective Review (Trock, *JAMA* 2008; DOI: 10.1001/jama.299.23.2760)

635 men with PSA >0.2 ng/mL post-RP. Retrospective review comparing no further treatment, salvage RT, and salvage RT with hormonal therapy (HT). Outcome was prostate cancer-specific survival (PCSS). Greatest benefit in PCSS if undetectable PSA after RT, doubling time <6 months, and PSA <2 ng/mL at time of salvage RT.

### American Urological Association/American Society for Radiation Oncology Guidelines on Adjuvant/Salvage Radiation After Prostatectomy (Thompson, *J Urol* 2013; DOI: 10.1016/j.juro.2013.05.032)

Guidelines for counseling patients to include appropriate indications for radiation in the adjuvant and salvage settings are presented.

# 34: BLADDER CANCER

*Rachit Kumar, MD*
*Deborah A. Kuban, MD*

## WORKUP

### All Cases
- H&P
- Urinalysis and cytology
- Cystoscopy with bladder mapping
- Transurethral resection of bladder tumor (TURBT) with random biopsies
- Imaging—CT chest/abdomen/pelvis, with IV contrast
- Labs—CBC, blood urea nitrogen (BUN), Creatinine, Alkaline Phosphatase

### Considerations
- Bone scan—if symptomatic or elevated alk phos

## TREATMENT RECOMMENDATIONS BY STAGE

| 0 (Ta or Tis) | TURBT alone → <br> (Adjuvant RT if persistently abnormal/equivocal cytology, multifocal disease, Gr 2/3, Tis/carcinoma in situ [CIS], T1 or subtotal resection) <br> OR TURBT + BCG × 6 weeks |
|---|---|
| I | TURBT → BCG × 6 weeks <br> (If disease persists >1 year, then cystectomy) <br> OR Bladder preservation chemoRT |
| II | Partial cystectomy (if involving only dome of the bladder) <br> OR Radical cystectomy/cystoprostatectomy <br> OR Bladder preservation with maximal TURBT → ChemoRT <br> OR Neoadjuvant chemotherapy → cystectomy |
| III | Radical cystectomy/cystoprostatectomy <br> OR Bladder preservation with maximal TURBT → ChemoRT <br> OR Neoadjuvant chemotherapy → cystectomy |
| IV | Chemotherapy <br> Palliative radiation |
| Locally recurrent | If bladder prior preservation treatment, then cystectomy <br> If prior cystectomy, then may consider local radiation |

## TECHNICAL CONSIDERATIONS

### Simulation
Simulate supine with two CT scans: bladder empty for initial whole bladder fields and bladder full for tumor boost

### Dose Prescription
*Definitive ChemoRT:*
- Initial fields to 45 Gy in 1.8 Gy/fx, boost to total dose of 60 to 66 Gy in 1.8 to 2 Gy/fx. Typically delivered with concurrent cisplatin, 20 to 40 mg/m$^2$ per week.

*Definitive RT:*
- Radiation alone should be considered palliative. Total dose is the same as noted in the preceding.
- Local recurrence after cystectomy:
  - Treat whole pelvis to 45 Gy in 1.8 Gy/fx and boost local recurrence up to 65 Gy 1.8 to 2 Gy/fx, depending on normal tissue tolerance.

### Target Delineation
- GTV = Area of initial tumor defined using multimodality evaluation (cystoscopy with bladder mapping, CT imaging)
- CTV initial fields = For initial fields treat entire bladder, prostatic urethra (in men), and draining nodes (obturator, internal and external iliacs) up to S2 to S3 (extend nodal coverage up to L5 to S1 when treating recurrence after cystectomy).
- CTV boost = Treat tumor bed/GTV. Some institutions use multiple cone downs to boost the bladder first then the tumor bed.
- PTV= Depends on treatment technique and daily imaging. Generally 2-cm margin on whole bladder and 7 mm around nodal drainage areas. 1- to 1.5-cm margin for boost area.

### Treatment Planning
- Treat initial fields with empty bladder. Boost volumes are treated with full bladder targeting known lesion as identified on bladder mapping and CT.
- Three-dimensional conformal radiation therapy (3DCRT) with 15- to 18-MV photons or intensity-modulated radiation therapy (IMRT) with 6-MV photons can be used. Daily imaging corresponding to technique, preferably cone beam CT.

## FOLLOW UP

- H&P every 3 months with urine cytology and cystoscopy × 1 year, then every 6 months × 2 years, then annually.
- CT abdomen/pelvis annually

## SELECTED STUDIES

### Massachusetts General Hospital Long-Term Outcomes—Bladder Preservation (Efstathiou, *Eur Urol* 2012; DOI: 10.1016/j.eururo.2011.11.010)

A report of 348 patients treated with the bladder-sparing technique at Massachusetts General Hospital (MGH) from 1986 to 2006. In appropriately selected patients, this approach provided results similar to cystectomy while preserving the bladder in >70% of patients.

### Pooled Analysis of Radiation Therapy Oncology Group Bladder-Preserving Trials (Mak, *J Clin Oncol* 2014; DOI: 10.1200/JCO.2014.57.5548)

Long-term outcome of six Radiation Therapy Oncology Group (RTOG) bladder-sparing trials are reported. Results were comparable to modern immediate cystectomy studies.

### Toxicity Related to Bladder-Sparing (Efstathiou, *J Clin Oncol* 2009; DOI: 10.1200/JCO.2008.19.5776)

Compiled toxicity related to RTOG bladder-sparing trials: 8903, 9506, 9706, and 9906. Seven percent late grade 3 pelvic toxicity: 6% GU, 2% GI, no grade 4.

### Bladder-Preservation With 2-Trimodality Techniques (Zapatero, *Urology* 2012; DOI: 10.1016/j.urology.2012.07.045)

Neoadjuvant methotrexate/cisplatin/vinblastine (MCV) followed by radiotherapy and weekly cis-Platinum with concurrent radiation produced similar outcomes although complete response and disease-free survival (DFS) were higher with the concurrent cis-Platinum-radiation approach.

### ICUD-EAU Guidelines on Muscle-invasive Bladder Cancer (Gakis, *Eur Urol* 2012; DOI: 10.1016/j.eururo.2012.08.009)

A comprehensive overview of radical cystectomy and bladder-sparing techniques in the treatment of muscle-invasive urothelial carcinoma of the bladder.

# 35: SEMINOMA
*Gary Walker, MD*
*Deborah A. Kuban, MD*

## WORKUP

### All Cases
- H&P, fertility
- Imaging—chest X-ray (CXR), testicular ultrasound, abdomen/pelvis CT
- Labs—alpha-fetoprotein (AFP), beta-human chorionic gonadotropin (beta-hCG), chemistry pre- and postorchiectomy

### Considerations
- CT chest if positive abdomen CT or abnormal CXR
- Sperm banking

## TREATMENT RECOMMENDATIONS BY STAGE

### After Radical Inguinal Orchiectomy

| IA, IB | Surveillance<br>OR Carbo one to two cycles<br>OR Para-aortic RT |
| --- | --- |
| IIA | Para-aortic/ipsilateral pelvic radiation RT<br>OR etoposide and cisplatin (EP) (four cycles)<br>OR bleomycin, etoposide, and cisplatin (BEP) (three cycles) |
| IIB | EP (four cycles)<br>OR BEP (three cycles) or Para-aortic/ipsilateral pelvic RT |
| IIC, III | EP (four cycles)<br>OR BEP (three cycles) |

## TECHNICAL CONSIDERATIONS

### Simulation
CT simulation supine. Clamshell to shield contralateral testicle

### Dose Prescription

- Stage I: 20 Gy in 2 Gy/fx to the para-aortics
- Stage II: 0 Gy in 2 Gy/fx to para-aortic and ipsilateral pelvic nodes, followed by a cone down to the gross disease to 30 Gy in 2 Gy/fx (Stage IIA) and 36 Gy in 2 Gy/fx (Stage IIB).

### Target Delineation

- Para-aortic anteroposterior/posteroanterior (AP/PA): Superior—bottom of T11, inferior bottom of L5, laterally cover transverse processes
- Stage II: Add an ipsilateral pelvic field to the para-aortic field with inferior boarder at the top of acetabulum.
- CT imaging should be used to assure coverage of nodal volumes at risk. Contour involved nodes.
- Cone Down: 1-cm margin on clinical target volume (CTV) (prescription isodose) with daily imaging.

Ipsilateral pelvic surgery such as herniorrhaphy or orchiopexy may alter lymphatic drainage; therefore, ipsilateral pelvic and inguinal radiation has been advocated. Chemotherapy may be considered as an alternative.

### Treatment Planning

- Three-dimensional conformal radiation therapy (3DCRT) AP/PA fields should be used. Intensity-modulated radiation therapy (IMRT) should be avoided to spare kidneys and reduce risk of second malignancy.
- >6-MV photons
- Right and left kidney D50% <8 Gy

### FOLLOW UP

#### After Orchiectomy Alone

- H&P q 3 to 6 months for 1 year, q 6 to 12 months for years 2 to 3 then annually
- CT abdomen/pelvis at 3, 6, 12 months, then q6 to 12 months for years 2 to 3 then q 12 to 24 months

#### After RT

- H&P q 6 to 12 months for 2 years, then annually
- CT abdomen/pelvis annually for 3 years

## SELECTED STUDIES

### Medical Research Council Optimal Target Volume Trial (Fossa, *J Clin Oncol* 1999; http://jco.ascopubs.org/content/17/4/1146.long)

A randomized trial of 478 patients treated from 1989 to 1993 with 30 Gy adjuvant radiation for Stage I seminoma to a para-aortic versus para-aortc + ipsilateral iliac field showed a relapse–free survival (RFS) of 96 % versus 97% with less toxicity.

### Medical Research Council TE 18—European Organization for Research and Treatment of Cancer 30942 (Jones, *J Clin Oncol* 2005; DOI: 10.1200/JCO.2014.59.1503)

A randomized trial of 625 patients treated from 1995 to 1998 with 30 Gy versus 20 Gy adjuvant radiation to a para-aortic field for Stage I seminoma showed that 20 Gy would not produce more than a 3% greater risk of relapse than 30 Gy with less morbidity.

### British Columbia (Kollmannsberger, *J Clin Oncol* 2015; DOI: 10.1200/JCO.2014.56.2116)

Retrospective review of 2483 patients with stage I seminoma and nonseminoma managed with surveillance. Low rates of relapse (13% in seminoma) with 5-yr disease-specific survival (DSS) of 99.7%.

### Medical Research Council TE19/ European Organization for Research and Treatment of Cancer 30982 (Oliver, *J Clin Oncol* 2011; DOI: 10.1200/JCO.2009.26.4655)

1447 patients with stage I randomized to one cycle carboplatin versus radiation (20 or 30 Gy in 2 Gy fractions to the para-aortic or para-aortic/ipsilateral pelvis). No difference in RFS but reduction in contralateral germ cell tumors with carboplatin (2% vs. 15%).

### German (Classen, *J Clin Oncol* 2003; DOI: 10.1200/JCO.2003.06.065)

94 patients treated with RT to para-aortic and high ipsilateral iliac LNs to a dose of 30 Gy (stage IIA) or 36 Gy (stage IIB). Excellent RFS at 6 years (stage IIA—95.3%, stage IIB—88.9%), with no late toxicity.

### Spanish Chemotherapy (Garcia-Del-Muro *J Clin Oncol* 2008; DOI: 10.1200/JCO.2007.15.9103)

72 patients with stage IIA or IIB treated with four cycles of EP or three cycles of BEP (nonrandomized). Excellent progression-free (90%) and overall survival (95%).

# 36: HODGKIN LYMPHOMA

*Neil Taunk, MD*
*Rahul R. Parikh, MD*

## WORKUP

### All Cases

- H&P (include weight change, performance status, constitutional symptoms, night sweats, pruritus, alcohol-induced pain)
- Imaging—PET/CT, chest X-ray (CXR)
- Labs—CBC, erythrocyte sedimentation rate (ESR), complete metabolic panel, albumin, lactate dehydrogenase (LDH), HIV test
- Biopsy—excisional lymph node biopsy preferred over core-needle biopsy

### If Stage III/IV or B-Symptoms

Bone marrow biopsy

## EARLY STAGE RISK GROUPING

| Study | Very High Risk | High Risk | Low Risk | Very Low Risk |
|---|---|---|---|---|
| German Hodgkin Study Group (GHSG) | | Mediastinal mass ratio >1/3 thorax; OR Extranodal disease; OR ≥3 nodal areas; OR ESR >50 (asymptomatic) OR ESR >30 (symptomatic) | No large mediastinal mass; AND No extranodal disease; AND <3 nodal areas; AND Low ESR | |
| European Organization for Research and Treatment of Cancer (EORTC) | | Age ≥50; OR ≥4 disease areas; OR Mediastinum thoracic ratio >0.35; OR ESR >50; OR ESR ≥30 with B symptoms | Age 40 to 49; OR Male; OR 2 to 3 disease sites; OR B symptoms and ESR <30 No high-risk features | Age <40; AND Female; AND Stage I; AND Mediastinum thoracic ratio <0.35; AND ESR <50; AND No B symptoms |

*(continued)*

| Study | Very High Risk | High Risk | Low Risk | Very Low Risk |
|-------|---------------|-----------|----------|---------------|
| National Cancer Information Center (NCIC) | Any lesion >10 cm; OR Mediastinal mass ratio ≥1/3 thorax; OR Intraabdominal disease | Age ≥40; OR ESR ≥50; OR Mixed cellularity or lymphocyte depleted histology; OR ≥4 disease areas No very high-risk features | Age <40; AND ESR <50; AND <4 disease sites; AND Nonmixed cellularity or lymphocyte depleted histology | <3 cm single cervical or epitrochlear node; AND Lymphocyte predominant or nodular sclerosing; AND ESR <50 |

## TREATMENT RECOMMENDATIONS BY STAGE

| I (favorable) | Chemo → Radiation<br>OR Chemo alone<br>OR RT alone (e.g. nodular lymphocyte-predominant Hodgkin lymphoma [NLPHL]) |
|---------------|-----------------------------------------------------------------------------------------------------------------------|
| IIA (favorable) | Chemo → Radiation<br>OR Chemo alone<br>OR RT alone (e.g., NLPHL) |
| I (unfavorable) | Chemo → Radiation<br>OR Chemo alone |
| II (unfavorable) | Chemo → Radiation<br>OR Chemo alone (proceed with caution) |
| IB, IIB | Chemo → Radiation |
| III | Chemo alone<br>OR Chemo ± Radiation (PET+ sites, initially bulky disease) |
| IV | Chemo alone<br>OR Chemo ± Radiation (PET +, initially bulky disease) |

## TECHNICAL CONSIDERATIONS

### Simulation

- Simulate supine with IV contrast and respiratory management (e.g., gating with deep inspiration breath hold [DIBH]) if appropriate for the site; arms up if treating axilla or arms akimbo if treating neck/supraclavicular fossa.
- Consider taping breast tissue out of RT field(s) when treating females.
- Consider pre-chemotherapy PET-CT simulation if available. Fuse pre-chemotherapy imaging to simulation scan.

**Dose Prescription**

- RT alone: 30 Gy involved-site RT (ISRT) in 1.8 to 2 Gy/fx (Consider 36 Gy for bulky lesions)
- Combined modality:
- Stage I to II, favorable: 20 Gy ISRT in 1.8 to 2 Gy/fx (only if meets GHSG criteria, i.e. HD10)
- Stage I to II, unfavorable: 30 Gy ISRT in 1.8 to 2 Gy/fx
- Stage I to II, bulky: 30 to 36 Gy ISRT in 1.8 to 2 Gy/fx
- Stage III to IV: 30 to 36 Gy in 1.8 to 2 Gy/fx

**Target Delineation**

- GTV based on pre- and post-chemotherapy imaging
- ITV = GTV with 4D motion assessment
- CTV = includes pre-chemotherapy GTV and ITV +1.0 to 1.5 cm, subtracting areas of low risk of clinical involvement (e.g. bone, muscle, air)
- PTV = CTV+ setup error 0.3 to 1.0 cm, based on treatment technique, site of disease, and use of daily imaging (e.g. three-dimensional conformal radiation therapy [3DCRT] vs. intensity-modulated radiation therapy [IMRT] with daily kV/cone-beam computed tomography [CBCT] imaging)

For additional target planning information please refer to:

- Modern radiation therapy for Hodgkin lymphoma: field and dose guidelines from the international lymphoma radiation oncology group (ILROG). Specht et al. *IJROBP* 2014

**Treatment Planning**

- 3D or IMRT (as appropriate for site)
- Consider Proton Beam Therapy in select cases to improve dose to OAR (e.g. kidney, heart, lung, breast)
- With heterogeneity corrections "on"

**FOLLOW UP**

- If asymptomatic:
  - H&P and labs every 3 to 6 months for years 1 and 2, then every 6 to 12 months until year 3, then annually. Thyroid stimulating hormone (TSH) every 6 months if RT to neck, upper mediastinum. CT after treatment once within 12 months, then as clinically indicated. Females start breast cancer screening 8 years after RT or age 40 (whichever is first) after mediastinal treatment

## SELECTED STUDIES

### HD4 (Duhmke, *J Clin Oncol* 2001; http://jco.ascopubs.org/content/19/11/2905.abstract)

376 Stage I to II patients without risk factors. No chemotherapy. All treated with involved-field radiotherapy (IFRT) 40 Gy then EFRT to 30 Gy versus 40 Gy. 7-year relapse-free survival (83% vs. 78%) and overall survival (OS) (96% vs. 91%) equivocal

### EORTC H8-F and H8-U (Ferme, *N Engl J Med* 2007; DOI: 10.1056/NEJMoa064601)

1538 patients with I to II supradiaphragmatic Hodgkin's lymphoma (HL), with favorable and unfavorable trials. H8-F compared MOPP-ABV × 3 + IFRT versus STNI. 5 year event-free survival (EFS) combined treatment 98% versus STNI 74% (SS). 10-year OS 97% versus 92% (SS). Recommend chemo ➔ IFRT

H8-U compared MOPP-ABV × 6 + IFRT versus MOPP-ABV × 4 + IFRT versus MOPP-ABV × 4 + STNI. 5-year EFS 84% versus 88% versus 87% (NS). 10-year OS 88% versus 85% versus 84% (NS). Recommend chemo × 4 ➔ IFRT

### HD7 (Engert, *J Clin Oncol* 2007; DOI: 10.1200/JCO.2006.07.0482)

650 IA-IIB HL patients without risk factors, randomized to RT ± ABVD × 2. RT was 30 Gy extended field radiation therapy (EFRT) + 10 Gy IFRT. 7-year disease-free survival (DFS) combined treatment 88% versus RT alone 67% (SS). 7-year OS combined treatment 94% versus RT alone 92% (NS). Combined modality therapy superior to RT alone

### HD10 (Engert, *N Engl J Med* 2010; DOI: 10.1056/NEJMoa1000067)

1131 patients stage I to II without risk factors randomized in 2 × 2 design to ABVD × 2 versus ABVD × 4, then IFRT 30 Gy versus IFRT 20 Gy. No significant difference in OS, freedom from treatment failure (FFTF), or progression-free survival (PFS). ABVD × 2 + 20 Gy IFRT standard for early-stage favorable HL.

### EORTC/GELA H10-F and H10-U (Raemaekers, *J Clin Oncol* 2014; DOI: 10.1200/JCO.2013.51.9298)

1137 patients with I/II supradiaphragmatic HL with favorable and unfavorable trials. Interim PET after two cycles for all arms.

H10-F randomized ABVD × 3 + INRT 30 Gy versus ABVD × 2 ➔ ABVD × 2 if PET(−), or BEACOPP × 2 + INRT 30 Gy if PET (+)

H10-U randomized ABVD × 4 + INRT 30 Gy versus ABVD × 2 ➔ ABVD × 4 if PET(−), or BEACOPP × 2 + INRT 30 Gy in PET(+)

Interim analysis showed combined modality treatment showed fewer early progressions

# 37: NON-HODGKIN LYMPHOMA

*Neil Taunk, MD*
*Rahul R. Parikh, MD*

## WORKUP

### All Cases
- H&P (include B-symptoms, splenomegaly)
- Imaging—CT C/A/P ± PET
- Labs—CBC, complete metabolic panel, LDH, HIV, Hepatitis B status
- Biopsy—excisional lymph node biopsy preferred over core-needle biopsy, immunophenotyping of specimen
- Bone marrow in most cases

### If Gastric MALT
- EGD with biopsy, *H. pylori*

### If Burkitt
- Lumbar puncture, HIV, Hep B/C

### If Extranodal NK/T-Cell Lymphoma (Nasal Type)
- EBV viral load

## TREATMENT RECOMMENDATIONS BY DISEASE AND STAGE

| CLL/SLL | I: Observe or radiation therapy (RT [palliation])<br>II–IV: Observe OR systemic therapy OR clinical trial OR transplant |
|---|---|
| Follicular lymphoma (Gr 1–2) | I–II: RT OR immunotherapy ± chemotherapy OR Observe<br>III–IV (asymptomatic): Observe<br>III–IV (symptomatic): chemo-immunotherapy OR palliative RT |
| Gastric MZL | I–II (*H. pylori* positive): antibiotic<br>I–II (*H. pylori* negative or t11:18 positive): RT<br>III–IV: Observe<br>III–IV (symptomatic): chemo-immunotherapy OR palliative RT |

(continued)

(continued)

| Nongastric MZL | I–II: RT or surgery OR immunotherapy OR observe (if asymptomatic)<br>IV: Manage as per stage IV follicular lymphoma |
|---|---|
| Mantle Cell | I–II: RT OR chemo ±RT<br>III–IV: Chemo |
| DLBCL | I–II: Chemo → RT OR chemo<br>IB, IIB: Chemo → ±RT<br>III–IV: Chemo → RT (bulky tumor or incomplete response) OR Chemo |
| PMBL/GZL | Chemo → RT<br>OR Chemo → ±RT |
| Burkitt Lymphoma | Chemo → ± palliative RT |
| AIDS-related B cell lymphomas | Burkitt: Chemo<br>DLBCL: Chemo<br>Plasmablastic: Chemo<br>PCNSL: Chemo OR palliative RT |
| ALCL (ALK+) | I–II: Chemo → RT OR chemo→ ±RT<br>III–IV: Chemo → ±RT |
| Other PTCL | Clinical Trial OR chemo → ±RT |
| Extranodal NK/T-cell (nasal type) | I: RT OR ChemoRT<br>I (with risk factors), II: ChemoRT<br>IV: ChemoRT OR clinical trial |
| Extranodal NK/T-cell (extranasal type) | I–IV: Clinical Trial OR chemoRT |

### TECHNICAL CONSIDERATIONS

#### Simulation

Site specific: simulate with IV/PO contrast and respiratory management (e.g., 4DCT for gastric MALT lymphoma or gating with DIBH for mediastinal disease) if appropriate; consider PET-CT simulation if available. Fuse prechemotherapy imaging to simulation scan.

#### Dose Prescription

- Indolent lymphomas (FL, MZL, SLL, and MCL)
- I to II: 20 to 30 Gy in 1.8 to 2 Gy/fx
- III/IV: 4 Gy in 2 Gy/fx local RT, repeat if needed for further palliation

- Aggressive lymphomas (DLBCL, PTCL)
  - CR after chemo: 30 to 39.6 Gy in 1.8 to 2 Gy/fx
  - PR after chemo: 40 to 50 Gy in 1.8 to 2 Gy/fx
  - Definitive (no chemo): 45 to 55 Gy in 1.8 to 2 Gy/fx
- PCNSL
  - CR after chemo: 23.4 to 24 Gy in 1.8 to 2 Gy/fx
  - PR after chemo: 36 to 45 Gy in 1.8 to 2 Gy/fx
  - Definitive (no chemo): 40 to 50 Gy in 1.8 to 2 Gy/fx
- Eye
  - Primary intraocular lymphoma: 36 Gy in 1.8 Gy/fx
  - Orbital: 24 to 30 Gy in 1.5 to 2 Gy/fx, Consider 4 Gy in 2 Gy/fx for palliation (may be repeated)
- Nasal Cavity and Paranasal Sinus
  - CR after chemo: 30 Gy in 1.8 to 2 Gy/fx
  - PR after chemo: 40 Gy in 1.8 to 2 Gy/fx
- Extranodal NK/T-cell
  - Concurrent ChemoRT: 50 Gy in 2 Gy/fx
  - Definitive: 50 Gy in 2 Gy/fx with 5 to 10 Gy in 1.8 to 2 Gy/fx boost
  - CR after chemo: 45 to 50 Gy in 1.8 to 2 Gy/fx
- Gastric MALT
  - Definitive: 30 Gy in 1.5 to 1.8 Gy/fx

**Target Delineation**
- GTV based on pre- and postchemotherapy imaging
- ITV = GTV with 4D motion assessment
- CTV = includes prechemotherapy GTV and ITV with 1.0- to 1.5-cm margin, subtracting areas of low clinical involvement (e.g., bone, muscle, and air)
- PTV = CTV+ setup error 0.3 to 1.0 cm, based on treatment technique, site of disease, and use of daily imaging (e.g., intensity-modulated radiation therapy [IMRT] with daily kV/CBCT imaging vs. conventional RT)

For additional target planning information please refer to:

- Modern radiation therapy for extranodal lymphomas: field and dose guidelines from the International Lymphoma Radiation Oncology Group. Yahalom et al. *IJROBP* 2015; DOI: 10.1016/j.ijrobp.2015.01.009
- Modern radiation therapy for nodal non-Hodgkin lymphoma-target definition and dose guidelines from the International Lymphoma Radiation Oncology Group. Illidge et al. *IJRBOP* 2014; DOI: 10.1016/j.ijrobp.2014.01.006

## Treatment Planning

- 3D or IMRT (as appropriate for site)
- Multi-field IMRT commonly used in Gastric MALT or head and neck cases to improve dose to OARs (e.g., kidney, heart, lungs, head and neck structures)
- May consider Proton Beam Therapy if OAR constraints do not meet preset criteria

## FOLLOW UP

- Site specific. If asymptomatic, generally clinical follow-up every 3 to 6 months up to 5 years, then annually or as clinically indicated
- MALT lymphoma: H&P every 3 to 6 months for 5 years, then as clinically indicated; if gastric, endoscopy every 6 months for 5 years, then annually
- FL (grade 1–2): H&P with labs every 3 to 6 months for 5 years; CT scan of site of disease no more than every 6 months up to 2 years
- DLBCL: H&P with labs every 3 to 6 months for 5 years; CT scan no more than every 6 months up to 2 years
- Burkitt: H&P with labs every 2 to 3 months for 1 year, then 3 months for 1 year, then every 6 months
- Extranodal NK/T-cell Lymphoma (nasal type): repeat initial imaging post-RT (e.g., CT, MRI, and PET-CT), endoscopy (annually) with visual biopsy, and EBV viral load

## SELECTED STUDIES

### FoRT (Hoskin, *Int J Radiat Oncol Biol Phys* 2012; DOI: 10.1016/j.ijrobp.2012.11.016)

Randomized noninferiority trial of FL/MZL requiring palliative or definitive treatment. Local progression-free survival (PFS) 93.7% (24 Gy) vs. 80.4% (4 Gy) without overall survival (OS) difference. Low-dose RT is effective in palliative setting, but inferior when radical treatment desired

### IELSG (Wirth, *Ann Oncology* 2013; DOI: 10.1093/annonc/mds623)

Retrospective multicenter trial of 102 patients (44 with relapsed disease) treated with median 40 Gy in 22 fractions. Fifteen-year freedom from treatment failure was 88% at median follow-up 7.9 years. RT alone has high cure rate in both primary and relapsed low-grade gastric MALT.

### MSKCC Gastric MALT Experience (Schechter, *J Clin Oncol* 1998; http://jco.ascopubs.org/content/16/5/1916.abstract)

Retrospective, 17 patients with I to II gastric MALT treated with median 30 Gy in 1.5 Gy fractions. 100% biopsy-confirmed complete response rate and 100% event-free survival at median 27 months.

### Korea Nasal-Type NK/T-Cell Lymphoma (Kim, *J Clin Oncol* 2009; DOI: 10.1200/JCO.2009.23.8592)

Phase II trial of 30 patients with IE-IIE nasal-type extranodal NK/T-cell lymphoma treated with median 40 Gy RT, concurrent weekly cisplatin, and adjuvant VIPD × 3. Three-year progression-free survival (PFS) 85% and OS 86%

### RTOG 9310 (DeAngelis, *J Clin Oncol* 2002; DOI: 10.1200/JCO.2002.11.013 and Fisher, *J Neurooncol* 2005; DOI: 10.1007/s11060-004-6596-9)

Phase II single arm of 98 HIV(−) patients. Preradiation MTX, vincristine, procarbazine, and intraventricular MTV → 45 Gy whole brain RT → high-dose cytabarine. If CR after induction, then WBRT 36 Gy BID. Median OS <60 years old 50.4 months; >60 years old 21.8 months. Fifteen percent with severe delayed neurotoxicity. Combined modality treatment superior to RT alone.

### ECOG 1484 (Horning, *J Clin Oncol* 2004; DOI: 10.1200/JCO.2004.06.088)

352 patients with Stage I with risk factors, IE, II, and IIE diffuse aggressive lymphomas randomized after CHOP × 8 to 30 Gy IFRT versus observation (40 Gy if PR). Ten-year OS 68% versus 65% (NS), but 6-year disease-free survival (DFS) 73% (RT) versus 56% (observation). Addition of low-dose RT improves local control.

### MDACC RCHOP + RT (Phan, *J Clin Oncol* 2010; DOI: 10.1200/JCO.2009.27.3441)

Retrospective. 469 patients with DLBCL (190 with Stage I or II disease). Seventy percent treated with at least six cycles RCHOP and 30.2% treated with 30 to 39.6 Gy IFRT. Matched-pair analysis showed patients with Stage I/II DLBCL receiving six to eight cycles of RCHOP and RT and improved OS and PFS compared to patients who did not receive RT.

# 38: MULTIPLE MYELOMA/ PLASMACYTOMA

*Jerry T. Liu, MD*
*Rahul R. Parikh, MD*

## WORKUP

### All Cases
- H&P
- Labs—CBC with differential, complete metabolic panel, LDH, beta-2-microglobulin, serum free monoclonal light chain (FLC), 24-hour urine protein, serum/urine protein electrophoresis, and immunofixation
- Imaging—Skeletal survey, if bone pain with negative XR or compression fracture: noncontrast CT, PET-CT, MRI
- Biopsy—unilateral bone marrow aspiration and biopsy with immunophenotyping, cytogenetics, and FISH analysis

### International Myeloma Working Group (IMWG) Criteria for Active (Symptomatic) Multiple Myeloma (MM)
(a) Clonal bone marrow plasma cells ≥10% or biopsy-proven plasmacytoma **and** (b) ≥1 of the following criteria: hypercalcemia, renal insufficiency, anemia, lytic bone lesion(s) on XR, CT, or PET-CT **or** ≥1 biomarker of malignancy:(≥60% clonal plasma cells, FLC ratio uninvolved:involved ≥100, >1 focal lesions on MRI)

### IMWG Criteria for Smoldering (Asymptomatic) MM
(a) serum M-protein ≥3 g/dL, urine M-protein ≥500 mg per 24 hour and/or 10% to 60% bone marrow plasma cells, (b) no myeloma-defining events or amyloidosis

### Criteria for Solitary Plasmacytoma (SP)
(a) biopsy proven single bone/soft tissue lesion, (b) normal bone marrow, (c) negative skeletal survey and MRI spine/pelvis, and (d) no anemia, hypercalcemia, and renal insufficiency

### Consideration for Bisphosphonate Therapy
Bone densitometry

### Consideration for Allogeneic Transplant
HLA typing

## TREATMENT RECOMMENDATIONS BY DISEASE AND STAGE

| SP | Bone: RT alone<br>Extramedullary: RT and/or surgery |
| --- | --- |
| Smoldering MM | Surveillance (3–6 m interval) |
| Active MM<br>(up to 40% cases will get RT) | Systemic therapy + bisphosphonate (evaluate response at two cycles) then consider for stem cell transplant<br>±RT ± surgery ± maintenance systemic therapy<br>RT indications: Uncontrolled pain, impending pathologic fracture, and cord compression |

## TECHNICAL CONSIDERATIONS

### Simulation
Immobilization and setup based on site of lesion. Wire superficial lesions + margin.

### Dose Prescription
*SP*
- RT ≥45 Gy in 1.8 to 2 Gy/fx (recent data suggest lower doses may be appropriate)

*MM*
- Single fraction (8 Gy) or RT 10 to 30 Gy in 2 to 5 Gy/fx, boost to ≥36 Gy for bulky disease, cord compression, or partial response. Commonly used prescription for palliation is 20 Gy in 10 fractions.

### Target Delineation
For vertebral SP or MM, consider covering one uninvolved body earlier and in the following.

*SP*
- GTV = visible lesion on all available imaging (e.g., MRI, PET-CT, pre-op scans)
- CTV = GTV + 2.0- to 3.0-cm margin (Elective nodal coverage for extramedullary SP should be considered)
- PTV = CTV + 0.3- to 0.5-cm setup error

*MM*

- Symptomatic lesion + margin, avoid uninvolved pelvic and long bones to preserve bone marrow.

## Treatment Planning

*SP*

- 3D, intensity-modulated radiation therapy (IMRT), or stereo-tactic body radiation therapy (SBRT) (based on site)

*MM*

- Typically opposed fields, more complex if needed
- Energy (6–10 MV) based on location

## FOLLOW UP

### SP

- Myeloma labs every 3 to 6 months, bone marrow aspirate and biopsy and imaging if indicated (>50% patients with bone SP progress to MM, <50% patients with extramedullary SP progress to MM)

### MM

- Myeloma labs every 3 months, skeletal survey annually or with symptoms, bone marrow aspirate and biopsy and imaging if indicated.

## SELECTED STUDIES

### Düsseldorf MM (Matuschek, *Radiat Oncol* 2015; DOI: 10.1186/s13014-015-0374-z)

Retrospective.107 patients with MM treated with palliative RT from 1989 to 2013. Median dose 25 Gy (range 8–50 Gy). Pain relief 85% (31% complete, 54% partial). Higher dose RT (30 Gy vs. 20 Gy) was associated with higher rate of pain relief and bone recalcification.

### Spinal Cord Compression MM (Rades, *Int J Radiat Oncol Biol Phys* 2006; DOI: 10.1016/j.ijrobp.2005.10.018)

Retrospective. International, multi-institutional.172 patients with MM treated with RT for SCC. 61 received short-course RT (8 Gy × 1, 4 Gy × 5) and 111 received long-course RT (3 Gy × 10, 2.5 Gy × 15, 2 Gy × 20). Median survival 17 months, LC 92%. More durable motor function improvement with long-course RT regimens, higher EQD2 (>30 Gy).

## MDACC SP (Reed, *Cancer* 2011; DOI: 10.1002/cncr.26031)

Retrospective. 84 patients with SP (59 bone, 25 extramedullary) treated with definitive RT from 1988 to 2008. Median dose 45 Gy (range 36–53.4 Gy). Five-year overall survival (OS) 78%, LC 92%, progression to MM 47%. Predictors of progression: bone site and serum protein at diagnosis. Seven patients had LR (two marginal, five in-field), no correlation with dose.

## Multicenter SP (Ozsahin, *Int J Radiat Oncol Biol Phys* 2006; DOI: 10.1016/j.ijrobp.2005.06.039)

Retrospective. 19 European and North American centers (Rare Cancer Network). 258 patients with SP (206 bone, 52 extramedullary) treated from 1977 to 2001, Median dose 40 Gy (range 20–66 Gy), no elective nodes treated. Five-year OS 74%, LC 86%, progression to MM 45%. Predictors for progression to MM: bone site. No dose-response for doses >30 Gy.

## Extramedullary SP (Alexiou, *Cancer* 1999; DOI: 10.1002/(SICI)1097-0142(19990601)85:11<2305:: AID-CNCR2>3.0.CO;2-3)

Literature Review. 869 patients with extramedullary SP (714 in upper aerodigestive tract [UAD] and 155 non-UAD) treated with either RT alone, surgery + RT, or surgery alone. Significantly higher OS and RFS with combined therapy for patients with UAD lesions. No survival difference between treatments for non-UAD lesions.

# 39: CUTANEOUS LYMPHOMA

*Neil Taunk, MD*
*Rahul R. Parikh, MD*

## WORKUP

### All Cases
- H&P (include total skin exam)
- Imaging—CT C/A/P ± PET/CT
- Labs—CBC, complete metabolic panel, LDH
- Biopsy—excisional, incisional, or punch biopsy with immunophenotyping and dermatopathology review

### If Rituximab to Be Considered
- Hepatitis B testing

### If Mycosis Fungoides (MF)/Sézary Syndrome
- Biopsy of suspicious lymph nodes, peripheral blood assessment for Sézary cells

## TREATMENT RECOMMENDATIONS BY DISEASE AND STAGE

| | |
|---|---|
| PCBCL(PCMZL/PCFCL) T1–T2 | RT OR excision OR topical therapy |
| PCBCL (PCMZL/PCFCL) T3 | Observation OR local RT OR topical therapy |
| DLBCL leg type | RCHOP ± local RT OR RT |
| PCTCL (ALCL) Localized | RT OR surgery ± RT |
| PCTCL (ALCL) Multifocal | RT OR systemic therapy OR observation |
| MF/Sézary syndrome IA–IIA: (localized) | RT OR topicals IA–IIA (generalized) TSEBT OR topicals |

*(continued)*

*(continued)*

| MF/Sézary syndrome IIB: (localized) | RT OR topicals; (generalized) systemic therapy |
| MF/Sézary syndrome III (no blood involvement) | TSEBT OR topicals |
| MF/Sézary syndrome III (blood involvement) | Systemic therapy ± RT |
| MF/Sézary syndrome IV | Systemic therapy ± RT |

## TECHNICAL CONSIDERATIONS

### Simulation

- Cutaneous lesions should be simulated with wire marking the lesion(s) with margin. Some local RT techniques may not require simulation (e.g., superficial RT).
- TSEBT treatment is often clinical setup.

### Dose Prescription

- PCMZL/PCFCL: 24 to 30 Gy in 1.8 to 2 Gy/fx
- Primary Cutaneous DLBCL, leg type: 36 to 40 Gy in 1.8 to 2 Gy/fx
- (40 Gy if no chemotherapy)
- PCTCL (ALCL): 24 to 36 Gy in 1.8 to 2 Gy/fx
- MF/Sézary: 20 to 24 Gy in 1.8 to 2 Gy/fx for local therapy
- For TSEBT 12 to 36 Gy in 1to 2 Gy/fx (daily, or twice per week if higher dose per fx)

### Target Delineation

- Contour or clinical setup
- GTV = visible or pre-excision/prechemotherapy lesion
- Clinical target volume (CTV) = includes GTV with 1.0- to 2.0-cm margin
- PTV = CTV + setup error 0.5 to 1.0 cm

For additional target planning information please refer to

- Modern Radiation Therapy for Primary Cutaneous LymphomasField and Dose Guidelines From the International Lymphoma Radiation Oncology Group
- Specht et al. *Int J Radiat Oncol Biol Phys* 2015; DOI: 10.1016/j.ijrobp.2015.01.008

### Treatment Planning

- 2D or 3D (as appropriate for site)
- Most superficial lesions can be completed with 6- or 9-MeV electrons with bolus (for sufficient skin dose) or superficial RT (e.g., 100 kV)
- Larger tumors may require opposed beams with bolus or megavoltage photon energy

TSEBT: Six-position large electron field technique (Stanford) with care to boost or supplement shielded areas including scalp, soles of feet, and perineum. Various techniques for electron beam degrading with goal Dmax at the skin surface, and 80% dose at 0.7- to 1.0-cm depth

### FOLLOW UP

If asymptomatic: H&P and labs every 3 to 6 months for years 1 and 2, then every 6 to 12 months until year 3, then annually. Patients must have total skin exam. TSH if appropriate every 6 months (e.g., patients who received TSEBT)

### SELECTED STUDIES

#### Yale (Smith, *J Clin Oncol* 2004; DOI: 10.1200/JCO.2004.08.044)

34 patients with PCBL treated with median 40 Gy radical RT (range 20–48 Gy). Sixty eight percent met WHO criteria for diffuse large cell subtype. Five-year LRFS 90% >36 Gy versus 50% <36 Gy. Leg-type had worse outcomes, suggesting a higher dose of radical RT required.

#### NCI MF (Kaye, *N Engl J Med* 1989; DOI: 10.1056/NEJM198912283212603)

103 patients with MF receiving 30 Gy TSEBT randomized to concurrent systemic chemotherapy or sequential topical therapy. Patients with combined treatment had higher complete response rate (38% vs. 18%), but no overall survival (OS) or disease-free survival (DFS) difference at median 75 months. Early aggressive concurrent treatment does not improve outcomes compared to conservative management with initial topical therapies.

### MDACC (Akhtari, *Leuk Lymph* 2015;
### DOI: 10.3109/10428194.2015.1040012)

Retrospective. 39 patients with 42 lesions indolent PCBCL. All achieved CR with radical radiotherapy. No difference in PFS in low dose (<12 Gy) versus high dose (>12 Gy) RT. All seven out-of-field relapses salvaged with RT. Recommend initial use of low-dose RT in radical treatment of these lesions.

### Stanford TSEBT (Navi, *JAMA Dermatol* 2011;
### DOI: 10.1001/archdermatol.2011.98)

Retrospective. 180 patients with MF treated from 1970 to 2007 treated with ≥ 30 Gy TSEBT ± topical nitrogen mustard. Hundred percent overall response rate with 60% achieving CR. Five-year OS 59% and 10-year OS 40%. Hundred percent overall response rate to patients receiving second course TSEBT.

# 40: SARCOMA

*Andrew Bishop, MD*
*B. Ashleigh Guadagnolo, MD*

## WORKUP

### All Cases
- H&P (consider presenting function and post-treatment function)
- MRI ± CT of primary lesion
- CT Chest
- Carefully planned biopsy (core needle or incisional)
- Pathologic confirmation of histologic subtype and grade
- Multidisciplinary evaluation at specialty center

### If Histologic Subtype Is Myxoid Liposarcoma
- CT Abd/Pelvis
- ±MRI total spine

### If Histologic Subtype Is Alveolar Soft Part Sarcoma
- MRI brain

## TREATMENT RECOMMENDATIONS OF SOFT TISSUE SARCOMA OF THE EXTREMITY/TRUNK/H&N BY STAGE

| | |
|---|---|
| IA (T1a-1b, G1)<br>IB (T2a-2b, G1) | Surgery alone with wide margins<br>If fail to obtain oncologic margins, consider re-resection or post-op RT<br>If tumor is located in location where surgical salvage would be morbid after recurrence (e.g., hands/feet, head, and neck region), consider pre-op RT then surgery as upfront treatment approach |
| IIA (T1a-1b, G2/G3), resectable | Surgery → RT<br>OR RT → Surgery<br>*wide excision alone should only be considered in select cases (e.g., superficial, wide margins possible) |
| IIB (T2a-2b, G2), resectable<br>III (T2a-2b, G3 or N1), resectable | Surgery → RT → ± chemo<br>OR RT → Surgery → ± chemo<br>OR chemo → RT → Surgery |
| II or III, unresectable | RT → Surgery → ±chemo<br>OR chemo → RT → Surgery |

*(continued)*

| Limited IV (oligo) | Treat primary per previously noted algorithms with chemo<br>For oligomets consider:<br>Metastasectomy<br>OR stereotactic body radiation therapy (SBRT)<br>OR ablative procedure |
| --- | --- |
| Disseminated IV | Palliation with chemo, RT, or surgery<br>OR supportive care |

## TREATMENT RECOMMENDATIONS FOR RETROPERITONEAL SARCOMAS

| Resectable | RT → Surgery → ±chemo<br>OR surgery ± IORT → ±chemo |
| --- | --- |
| Unresectable | Attempt cytoreduction with combination chemoRT, then reconsider surgical options.<br>OR palliative care |

## TREATMENT RECOMMENDATIONS FOR DESMOID TUMORS

| Resectable | Observation<br>OR surgery<br>OR RT<br>OR systemic therapy |
| --- | --- |
| Unresectable | RT<br>OR systemic therapy<br>OR observation |

## TECHNICAL CONSIDERATIONS

### Simulation

Simulate with considerations depending on primary site (e.g., for extremities ensure rotational immobilization by anchoring foot/hand)

### Dose Prescription

*Soft Tissue Sarcomas of Extremities/Trunk/H&N*

- Pre-op RT: 50 Gy in 2 Gy/fx external beam radiation therapy (EBRT)
- In case of an R1 resection could consider post-op EBRT boost 16 to 18 Gy in 2 Gy/fx OR brachytherapy 14 to 16 Gy in 3 to 4 Gy/fx BID or IORT 10 to 12.5 Gy boost

- Post-op RT: 50 Gy in 2 Gy/fx EBRT with cone-down boost 10 to 18 in 2 Gy/fx Gy depending on margin status

*Desmoid*
- RT alone: 56 to 58 Gy in 2 Gy/fx

## Target Delineation
- Consider fusing pre and/or post-op MR imaging with planning CT for better target delineation
- Consider anatomic compartments, joints, and bones when delineating targets

*Pre-Op*
- Careful evaluation of contrast-enhanced T1-weighted MRI for extent of disease
- GTV = Based on imaging (include T1 + contrast tumor but not peritumoral edema seen on T2)
- CTV = 3.5- to 4-cm expansion in longitudinal direction, 1.5-cm radial expansion (ensuring peritumoral edema is included in CTV)
- PTV = 1-cm isotropic expansion

*Post-Op*
Discuss margins with surgeon

- GTV = Recreate pre-op tumor to identify tumor extensions
- *Elective* CTV = 3.5- to 4-cm expansion in longitudinal direction with 1.5 cm radially, ensuring coverage of surgical bed and clips
- *Boost* CTV = 2-cm expansion on reconstructed GTV with 1.5 cm radially
- PTV = 1-cm isotropic expansion on both CTV volumes

## Treatment Planning
- 6- to 18-MV photons
- Often 3D plans are used in extremities
- Intensity-modulated radiation therapy (IMRT) useful in certain scenarios and may improve LC or reduce fracture risk
- Consider bolus for superficial lesions

## FOLLOW UP

- Eval for rehab or PT until maximal function achieved
- H&P q3 to 6 months × 2 to 3 years then annually
- Chest imaging (CT or plain film) 3 to 6 months for 2 to 3 years then q6 months for 2 years, then annually.
- MRI or CT of primary site q3 to 6 months for 2 to 3 years, then q6 months for 2 years through 5 years of surveillance.

## SELECTED STUDIES

### The Treatment of Soft-Tissue Sarcomas of the Extremities: Prospective Randomized Evaluations (Rosenberg, *Ann Surg* 1982; http://www.ncbi.nlm.nih.gov/pmc/articles/PMC1352604/)

Randomized patients with STS of the extremity to amputation versus limb-sparing surgery and radiation. Outcomes related to LC, disease-free survival (DFS), and overall survival (OS) were equivalent, making limb-sparing surgery with RT the standard of care.

### Randomized Prospective Study of the Benefit of Adjuvant Radiation Therapy in the Treatment of STS of the Extremity (Yang, *J Clin Oncol* 1998; http://jco.ascopubs.org/content/16/1/197.abstract)

Randomized patients post limb-sparing surgery ± post-op RT. Patients receiving post-op RT had improved LC but resulted in worse limb strength, edema, and range of motion.

### Pre-Op versus Post-Op RT in STS of the Limbs: A Randomized Trial (O'Sullivan, *Lancet* 2002; DOI: 10.1016/S0140-6736(02)09292-9)

Randomized patients with STS to pre-op RT (50 Gy) versus post-op RT (66 Gy) and showed equivalent disease control. However, pre-op RT resulted in higher rates of wound complications and post-op RT resulted in more late complications (extremity function).

### Comparison of Local Recurrence With Conventional and IMRT for Primary STS of the Extremity (Folkert, *J Clin Oncol* 2014; DOI: 10.1200/JCO.2013.53.9452)

Retrospectively reviewed patients with STS of the extremity treated with IMRT versus conventional EBRT. IMRT was independently associated with reduced LR on MV analysis (HR 0.46, $P = .02$)

**RTOG Contouring Consensus (Wang, *Int J Radiat Oncol Biol Phys*, 2011; DOI: 10.1016/j.ijrobp.2011.04.038) and Review of RT for Extremity STS (Haas, *Int J Radiat Oncol Biol Phys* 2012; DOI: 10.1016/j.ijrobp.2012.01.062)**

These two studies give consensus recommendations on contouring. They were incorporated into the summary found within this chapter.

**Treatment Guidelines for Pre-Op Radiation Therapy for Retroperitoneal Sarcoma: Preliminary Consensus of an International Expert Panel (Baldini, *Int J Radiat Oncol Biol Phys* 2015; DOI: 10.1016/j.ijrobp.2015.02.013)**

International expert consensus report on guidelines for pre-op RT for retroperitoneal sarcomas.

# 41: NON MELANOMA SKIN CANCER

*Anna Likhacheva, MD*

## WORKUP

### All Cases

- H&P (complete skin exam)
- Imaging—CT/MRI/PET when clinically indicated

### Considerations

- Radiation therapy is contraindicated in genetic conditions predisposing to skin cancer (e.g., basal cell nevus syndrome, xeroderma pigmentosum). Increased risks of adverse effects in areas prone to repeated trauma or poor circulation (e.g., belt line, feet, and pretibial skin). H (mask area), M (cheek, forehead, scalp, neck, pretibial), L (trunk and extremities) areas have varying risks of local recurrence.

## TREATMENT RECOMMENDATIONS BY STAGE

| | |
|---|---|
| T1/T2 operable | Surgery (WLE, Mohs micrographic) → RT for high risk[a] or positive margins<br>Nodal management if N+ or high risk of nodal involvment |
| T1/T2 inoperable | RT to primary (topical/destructive therapies for superficial lesions are an option)<br>Nodal management if N+ or high risk of nodal involvement |
| Nodal management:<br>cN0 but risk >15% (e.g., G3, PNI) | Elective dissection<br>OR elective RT |
| Nodal management:<br>cN+ or pN+<br>operable | Therapeutic dissection → consider adjuvant RT if multiple nodes positive, ECE, or cervical node(s) involved. Consider adjuvant chemoRT if cervical nodes with ECE |
| Nodal management:<br>cN+ or pN+<br>inoperable | RT ± concurrent chemotherapy |
| M1 | Cisplatin ± 5FU, and EGFR inhibitors<br>Clinical trial |

[a]High risk features for SCC: >2-mm thickness, Clarke level ≥4, PNI, primary site (ears, nonhair-bearing lip), and poor differentiation

## TECHNICAL CONSIDERATIONS

### Simulation

CT simulation for most definitive cases, intensity-modulated radiation therapy (IMRT), and previous RT. Clinical set up is an option for orthovoltage treatment, skin surface brachytherapy, small lesions, or palliative cases.

- Use bolus of appropriate thickness to bring dose to surface.
- Skin collimation should be used for electron field sizes <4 cm. Skin collimation encouraged for lesions near the eyes and nose where lateral constriction of isodose can be an issue.
- Radioopaque wire to outline lesion and CTV.
- IMRT planning for named nerve involvement coverage to skull base.

### Dose Prescription

*Definitive RT*

- For most lesions and optimal cosmesis: 66 Gy in 33 fx or 55 Gy in 20 fx delivered daily.
- For <2-cm lesions or palliation of large lesions: 50 Gy in 15 fx, 40 Gy in 10 fx, 35 Gy in 5 fx delivered daily.
- Skin surface brachytherapy: 40 Gy in 8 fx; 44 Gy in 10 fx delivered twice or thrice per week, at least 48 hour apart.
- Nodal areas that are clinical negative but at significant risk: 50 Gy in 25 fx.

*Adjuvant RT to Primary Site*

- 60 Gy in 30 fx or 50 Gy in 20 fx delivered daily

*Adjuvant RT to Regional Nodes*

- With ECE: 60 to 66 Gy in 30 to 33 fx (2 Gy/fx)
- Without ECE: 56 to 60 Gy in 28 to 30 fx (2 Gy/fx)

### Target Delineation

*Lesion Size and Histology Guide Optimal CTV Margin*

- 1 to 1.5 cm for <2-cm primary tumors
- 1.5 to 2 cm for >2-cm primary tumors, high risk squamous cell carcinoma, infiltrative basal cell carcinoma.

### Treatment Planning

- Electron beam therapy is the most common delivery method. If skin collimation is used, it should be modeled correctly in planning software. Electron beam doses are typically specified at 90% of the maximal depth dose (Dmax). Appropriate beam energy should deliver adequate surface dose and encompass the deep margin of the tumor by at least the distal 90% line.

- Orthovoltage x-ray doses are specified at Dmax (skin surface) to account for the relative biologic difference between the two modalities of radiation.
- IMRT can be used for large skin targets or for nodal irradiation.
- Bolus is necessary to achieve adequate skin surface dose with electron beam and IMRT.

## FOLLOW UP

- BCC: H&P, complete skin exam q6 to 12 months for life
- SCC localized: H&P q3 to 12 months for 2 years, then q6 to 12 months for 3 years, then q1 year for life
- SCC regional: H&P q1 to 3 months for year 1, then q2 to 4 months for year 2, then q4 to 6 months for years 3 to 5, then q6 to 12 months for life

## SELECTED STUDIES

### MDACC (Clayman et al., *J Clin Oncol* 2005)

Prospectively enrolled 210 patients with cutaneous SCC. Study showed a reduction in disease-specific survival (DSS) in patients with local recurrence at presentation, increasing size and depth, invasion beyond subcutaneous tissues, and PNI. Patients with > one risk factor compared with no risk factors had a significantly inferior 3-year DSS (70% vs. 100%).

### CTV Margins in Radiotherapy Planning for NMSC (Khan, *Radiother Oncol* 2012; DOI: 10.1016/j.radonc.2012.06.013)

A prospective, single arm, study of 159 patients with 150 lesions. The distance of microscopic tumor extension beyond a gross lesion varied from 1 mm to 15 mm, with a mean of 5.3 mm. The microscopic tumor extent was positively correlated with the size of gross lesion, and histology. Recommended CTV margins: 10 mm for BCC less than 2 cm, 13 mm for BCC greater than 2 cm, 11 mm for SCC less than 2 cm, and 14 mm for SCC greater than 2 cm.

### Radiotherapy for Epithelial Skin Cancer (Locke, *Int J Radiat Oncol Biol Phys* 2001)

Retrospective study of 468 patients with 531 lesions showed the following control rate with RT alone: basal cell was 95% (86% if recurrent), 89% for squamous cell (68% if recurrent). For basal cell, improved control with larger fraction size (>2 Gy).

# 42: MALIGNANT MELANOMA

*Anna Likhacheva, MD*

## WORKUP

### All Cases
- H&P (complete skin exam)
- Imaging—CT/MRI/PET for specific signs or symptoms or stage ≥III (LN+)

### Considerations

ABCDE (asymmetry, borders, color, diameter, and enlargement). Full thickness biopsy rather than shave.

## TREATMENT RECOMMENDATIONS BY STAGE

| Stage IA–IIC | Wide local excision (WLE) with minimum 1- to 2-cm margins. Sentinel node biopsy (SLNBx) for ulceration or >0.75- to 1-mm thick → Post-op RT to primary site for desmoplastic melanoma, extensive PNI or locally recurrent disease → may consider interferon alpha for stage IIB–IIC |
|---|---|
| Stage III | WLE and SLNBx → Lymph node dissection → Post-op RT to primary site for desmoplastic melanoma, extensive PNI or locally recurrent disease. Post-op RT to a nodal basin for high-risk features* → systemic treatment with Interferon alpha, or high-dose ipilimumab, or biochemotherapy |
| Stage IV | Anti-PD1 therapy, targeted therapy if BRAF mutated, intralesional therapy, biochemotherapy. |

*High-risk features: ECE, ≥1 parotid LN, ≥2 cervical/axillary LN, ≥3 inguinal LN, cervical LN ≥3 cm in size, axillary/groin LN ≥4 cm in size.

## TECHNICAL CONSIDERATIONS

### Simulation

Set up and technique vary with the site of primary lesion. CT simulation. Use bolus of appropriate thickness to bring dose to surface. Radioopaque wire to outline scars.

## Dose Prescription
Clinical practice fraction size varies. Some regimens influenced by radiobiological experiments suggesting that melanoma radiosensitivity is directly proportional to fraction size.

- 48 Gy in 2.4 Gy/fx was used in the randomized TROG trial. (Max dose to spine and brain is 40 Gy.)
- 30 Gy in 6 Gy/fx delivered biweekly over 2.5 weeks. (Max dose to spinal cord, brain, bowel, or brachial plexus should not exceed 24 Gy. Diligent dosimetry and set up are essential for this fractionation because dose inhomogeneity is exaggerated. Acceptable coverage of the targeted region when using photons is the 27 Gy isodose line.)

## Target Delineation
For adjuvant radiation of the primary site, the target is post-op bed + 2-cm margin for CTV.

For nodal radiation, the target is ipsilateral draining lymphatics.

- Cervical region—can use neutral or open-neck position. For latter, use appositional electron fields (bolus is used to limit the dose to the temporal lobe and the larynx).
- Axilla—axillary nodes only. No need to target supraclavicular nodes unless involved.
- Inguinal—usually less comprehensive than targets for the cervical and axillary regions, to minimize the risk of morbid lymphedema. No need to target external or common iliac nodal chains unless involved.

## Treatment Planning
Bolus is necessary to achieve adequate skin surface dose

## FOLLOW UP
- Annual skin exam for life (all stages)
- For stages IA to IIA: H&P q3 to 12 months for 5 years, then annually; routine labs/imaging not recommended
- For stages IIB to IV: H&P q3 to 6 months for 2 years, then q3 to 12 months for 3 years, then annually; routine labs for first 5 years; consider imaging.

## SELECTED STUDIES

### ANZNTG 01.02/TROG 02.01 (Henderson, *Lancet Oncol* 2015; DOI: 10.1016/S1470-2045(15)00187-4)

Randomized trial of 217 patients: observation versus lymph-node field RT in patients with high risk features. 48 Gy in 20 fx. No difference in overall survival (OS) or RFS at 73 months median f/u. SS improved LRC (HR 0.52.) Increased risk of lower extremity lymphedema in RT group (15% vs. 7.7%.) No difference in lymphedema for upper extremity.

### MDACC Experience (Ballo, *Cancer* 2003)

Retrospective review of 160 patients with cervical LN mets from melanoma. Median dose of 30 Gy at 6 Gy per fraction delivered twice weekly. Adjuvant radiotherapy resulted in a 10-year regional control rate of 94%.

### Fractionation for Malignant Melanoma (Chang, *Int J Radiat Oncol Biol Phys* 2006)

Retrospective study of 56 patients. Post-op RT provides excellent locoregional control and distant metastases is the main cause of mortality. Hypofractionation and conventional fractionation are equally efficacious.

### RT for Desmoplastic Melanoma (Guadagnolo, *Cancer* 2014; DOI: 10.1002/cncr.28415)

Retrospective review of 130 patients with desmoplastic melanoma. LR without post-op RT was 24%, while 7% with post-op RT.

### RT for Axillary Metastases (Beadle, *Int J Radiat Oncol Biol Phys* 2009; DOI: 10.1016/j.ijrobp.2008.06.1910)

Retrospective analysis of 200 patients with axillary metastases. 95 patients (48%) received RT to the axilla only and 105 patients (52%) to the axilla and supraclavicular fossa (EF). RT to the axilla only produced equivalent LR control to EF and resulted in lower treatment-related complications.

### RTOG 83-05 (Sause, *Int J Radiat Oncol Biol Phys* 1991)

Randomized trial of 126 patients: 32 Gy in 4 weekly fx versus 50 Gy in 20 daily fx. No difference between the arms.

# 43: MERKEL CELL CARCINOMA

*Anna Likhacheva, MD*

## WORKUP

### All Cases

- H&P (complete skin exam, lymph node exam)
- Imaging—PET/CT/MRI when clinically indicated

### Considerations

Merkel cell carcinoma has a high rate of local-regional relapse after surgery, is radiosensitive, and has poor prognosis. Although, RT is typically delivered in post-op setting, RT to primary site and undissected neck can be considered. Rates of occult and clinically evident nodal metastases at presentation are 30% to 50% and 20% to 25%, respectively.

## TREATMENT RECOMMENDATIONS BY STAGE

| T1/T2 operable | Wide local excision (WLE) with minimum 1- to 2-cm margins or MOHS with sentinel node biopsy (SLNBx)<br>Adjuvant RT for close margins, >1-cm tumors, lymphovascular invasion, immunosuppression |
|---|---|
| T1/T2 inoperable | RT to primary |
| cN0 | SLNBx or elective dissection or elective RT |
| cN+ or pN+ | Therapeutic dissection and/or combined radical RT to primary site and nodal basin |

## TECHNICAL CONSIDERATIONS

### Simulation

*CT Simulation*

- Use bolus of appropriate thickness to bring dose to surface.
- Radioopaque wire to outline lesion, scars and 5-cm CTV expansion.

### Dose Prescription

- RT doses are generally lower for MCC than for squamous and basal cell carcinoma because of increased radiosensitivity.
- Definitive RT: 60 to 66 Gy in 2 Gy/fx

- Microscopic disease: 56 to 60 Gy in 2 Gy/fx
- Clear margins: 46 to 56 Gy in 2 Gy/fx
- Elective nodal RT: 46 to 50 Gy in 2 Gy/fx

**Target Delineation**

- Wide margins (5 cm) should be used, if possible, around the primary site. Margins for boost volume is 1 to 2 cm. For head and neck primary, all ipsilateral cervical nodal levels may be included. If the primary site and nodal basin are being irradiated, treated contiguously when feasible.

**Treatment Planning**

- Electron beam therapy if simple superficial target. If skin collimation is used, it should be modeled correctly in planning software. Electron beam doses are typically specified at 90% of the maximal depth dose (Dmax). Appropriate beam energy should deliver adequate surface dose and encompass the deep margin of the tumor by at least the distal 90% line.
- Orthovoltage x-ray doses are specified at Dmax (skin surface) to account for the relative biologic difference between the two modalities of radiation.
- Intensity-modulated radiation therapy (IMRT) can be used for large skin targets or for nodal irradiation.
- Bolus is necessary to achieve adequate skin surface dose with electron beam and IMRT.

**FOLLOW UP**

H&P, complete skin and lymph node exam q3 to 6 months for 2 years, then q6 to 12 months for life. Consider routine imaging for high risk patients.

**SELECTED STUDIES**

**MDACC (Bishop, *Head Neck* 2015; DOI: 10.1002/hed.24017)**
Retrospective review of 106 patients with MCC of head and neck. No regional recurrences in 22 patients treated with RT to gross nodal disease without neck dissection. Lymphadenopathy at presentation impacted distant metastatic-free survival outcomes ($P < .001$).

### SEER Analysis (Mojica, *J Clin Oncol* 2007)

Survey of 1,665 cases of MCC in the SEER registry. The use of adjuvant radiation therapy is associated with improved survival in patients with MCC.

### Effect of RT Dose and Volume on Relapse in MCC (Foote, *Int J Radiat Oncol Biol Phys* 2010; DOI: 10.1016/j.ijrobp.2009.05.067)

Retrospective analysis of 112 patients. The in-field relapse rate was 3% for primary disease, and relapse was significantly lower for patients receiving >50 Gy.

### Features Predicting Sentinel Node Positivity in MCC (Schwartz, *J Clin Oncol* 2011; DOI: 10.1200/JCO.2010.33.4136)

Retrospective analysis of 95 patients. Increasing clinical size, increasing tumor thickness, increasing mitotic rate, and infiltrative tumor growth pattern were significantly associated with a greater likelihood of a positive SLNBx.

### TROG 96:07 (Poulsen, *J Clin Oncol* 2003)

Phase 2 study of 53 patients with high risk nonmetastatic MCC (recurrence after initial therapy, involved nodes, primary tumor size >1 cm, gross residual disease after surgery, or occult primary with nodes.) Treatment consisted of 50 Gy in 25 fractions with concurrent etoposide. The 3-year OS, LRC, and DC were 76%, 75%, and 76%, respectively. Tumor site and the presence of nodes were factors that were predictive for local control and survival. Multivariate analysis indicated that the major factor influencing survival was the presence of nodes.

# 44: EPENDYMOMA

*James Y. Rao, MD*
*Sahaja Acharya, MD*
*Stephanie M. Perkins, MD*

## WORKUP

### All Cases
- H&P
- MRI brain (pre-op and <48 hours post-op)
- MRI spine 10 to 14 days after surgery to avoid false+
- CSF cytology 10 to 14 days after surgery to avoid false+
- CBC, CMP

### Considerations
- Avoid presurgical LP if concern for hydrocephalus
- Gross total resection is most important prognostic factor, consider second surgery in setting of subtotal resection

## TREATMENT RECOMMENDATIONS

| | |
|---|---|
| Resectable tumor, Gross total resection, WHO Grade II and Supratentorial location | Maximum safe resection<br>Adjuvant RT to tumor bed, observation being studied on prospective clinical trial |
| Resectable tumor, Gross total resection, All others | Maximum safe resection<br>Adjuvant RT to tumor bed |
| Resectable tumor, Subtotal resection | Maximum safe resection<br>Consider chemo and second-look surgery<br>Adjuvant RT to tumor bed |
| Unresectable tumor | Definitive radiation to tumor |
| +LP or +MRI spine | Maximum safe resection<br>Craniospinal irradiation<br>RT boost to tumor bed<br>RT boost to gross spine disease |
| Recurrent tumor | Maximum safe resection<br>Consider reirradiation<br>Consider chemotherapy |

## TECHNICAL CONSIDERATIONS

### Simulation

Simulate and treat with thermoplastic mask, and anesthesia if necessary. Fuse pre- and postsurgical MRI to aid planning. If large resection cavity, repeating brain MRI at time of simulation is reasonable as cavity may contract significantly in size.

### Dose Prescription

- Adjuvant RT to Tumor Bed: 54 to 59.4 Gy in 1.8 Gy/fx
- Definitive RT: 54 to 59.4 Gy in 1.8 Gy/fx
- +LP or +MRI Spine: CSI 36 Gy, tumor bed 54 to 59.4 Gy, gross spinal disease 45 Gy all in in 1.8 Gy/fx
- Children <18 months with GTR recommend 54 Gy in 1.8 Gy/fx to tumor bed

### Target Delineation

- Contour based on post-op MRI and sim CT
- Tumor extent on pre-op imaging should be considered as well but tumor bed contour is primarily based on post-op imaging
- GTV = Tumor bed and residual disease
- Clinical target volume (CTV) = GTV + 10 mm, anatomically confined expansion
- PTV = CTV + 3 to 5 mm
- CTV/PTV expansions may extend into the brainstem
- If treating to 59.4 Gy, consider cone down boost after 54 Gy to limit brainstem dose.
- Limit dose to the spinal cord (54 Gy) and optic chiasm (50.4–54 Gy)

### Treatment Planning

- Consider proton beam radiation
- Intensity-modulated radiation therapy (IMRT) may reduce dose to hippocampus or cochlea compared to 3DCRT depending on location of tumor
- Daily imaging (2D:2D) to decrease PTV margins

## FOLLOW UP

If asymptomatic: H&P with MRI brain every 4 months for 3 years, then every 6 months for 2 more years, then every 6 to 12 months. MRI spine every year for first 5 years. See ACNS0831 FU schedule.

## SELECTED STUDIES

### ACNS0121 (Merchant, *Lancet Oncol* 2009; DOI: 10.1016/S1470-2045(08)70342-5)

Phase II study 153 patients, majority treated with 59.4 Gy after surgery. Seven-year local control, EFS, and overall survival (OS) were 88·7%, 76·9%, and 85·0%. OS influenced by grade and extent of resection.

### ACNS0121 Neurocognitive Outcomes (Merchant, *J Clin Oncol* 2004; DOI: 10.1200/JCO.2004.11.142)

Neurocognitive outcomes of 88 patients treated on ACNS0121 were stable and within normal limits, with more than half of cohort tested at or beyond 24 months.

### MGH Proton Therapy Experience (MacDonald, *Neuro Oncol* 2013; DOI: 10.1093/neuonc/not121)

70 children treated with proton beam to the tumor bed between 2000 and 2011. Three-year local control, progression-free survival (PFS), and OS of 83%, 76%, and 95%, respectively.

# 45: MEDULLOBLASTOMA

*James Y. Rao, MD*
*Sahaja Acharya, MD*
*Stephanie M. Perkins, MD*

## WORKUP

### All Cases

- H&P
- MRI brain (pre-op and <48 hours post-op)
- MRI spine 10 to 14 days after surgery to avoid false+
- CSF cytology 10 to 14 days after surgery to avoid false+
- CBC, CMP

### Considerations

- Avoid presurgical LP if concern for hydrocephalus
- VP shunt needed for ~30% of patients
- Posterior fossa syndrome can develop 12 to 24 hours post-op: p/w mutism, truncal ataxia, dysphagia. Do not delay RT.
- Baseline audiometry, IQ testing, TSH and growth measures
- M stage is the most important prognostic clinical factor
- Genetic subtypes: WNT (best prognosis), SHH, Group 3 (worst prognosis), Group 4

## TREATMENT RECOMMENDATIONS

| Standard Risk Age>3 years and <1.5 cm² residual and M0 | Maximal safe resection → CSI and posterior fossa boost with concurrent vincristine → Chemo |
| --- | --- |
| High Risk: >1.5 cm² residual OR M+ | Maximal safe resection → CSI and posterior fossa boost and boost to metastatic sites with concurrent vincristine → Chemo |
| High Risk: Age <3 years | Maximal safe resection → Chemo until 3 y/o → CSI and posterior fossa boost<br>If GTR + desmoplastic histology, can consider omitting RT |

## TECHNICAL CONSIDERATIONS

### Simulation

Simulate supine or prone with neck extended (PA spine field does not exit through oral cavity), shoulders positioned inferiorly (to allow for feathering of the spine and cranial field junctions) with thermoplastic mask, and anesthesia if necessary. Fuse post-surgical MRI to aid planning.

## Dose Prescription

- Standard risk: CSI 23.4 Gy in 1.8 Gy/fx, PF boost on conformal tumor bed boost to 54 Gy 1.8 Gy/fx
- High risk: CSI 36 Gy in 1.8 Gy/fx, PF boost to 55.8 Gy, boost intracianial or spinal metastases 39.6–50.4 Gy depending on location (refer to ACNS 0332)

## Target Delineation

*PA Spine Field (Plan First)*

- Superior extent: right above the shoulders, Inferior extent: thecal sac (usually at S2–S3), Lateral extent: 1-cm lateral to vertebral body and including the sacral nerve roots inferiorly.

*Cranial Field With Opposed Laterals*

- Rotate the collimator to match the divergence of the spine field (Collimator angle = arc $\tan^{-1}[0.5 \times$ spine field length/SSD])
- Kick the couch toward the gantry to avoid divergence of the cranial field into the spine field.
- (Couch kick angle = arc $\tan^{-1}[0.5 \times$ cranial field length/SAD])
- PF: Contour PF based on post-op MRI and sim CT
- Inferior extent: C1, Superior extent: Tentorium (best visualized on MRI), Lateral extent: Temporal bones and occiput Anterior: anterior brainstem
- CTV = PF (as described previously)
- PTV = CTV + 3 to 5 mm
- Refer to ACNS 0331 for contouring guidelines and atlas.

## Treatment Planning

- Consider proton beam radiation for CSI
- At Washington University, the junctions are feathered (shift in 1.0 cm) every 5 fractions. Purpose of feathering junction is to avoid hot/cold spots.
- Organs at risk: brainstem (max <56 Gy), optic chiasm (max < 54 Gy), cochlea, pituitary gland, and hypothalamus.
- CBC should be obtained weekly while undergoing CSI

## FOLLOW UP

- If asymptomatic: H&P with MRI brain every 3 to 6 months for 2 years, then every 6 months for 2 more years, then every 6 to 12 months. MRI spine every 4 to 6 months for 2 years, then every year for 2 more years.
- Regular exams to monitor treatment sequelae: neurocognitive evaluation, neuropsychiatric evaluation, neuroendocrine evaluation, and audiology exam. Be cognizant of secondary malignancies.

## SELECTED STUDIES

### SFOP M4 (Bouffet, *Int J Radiat Oncol Biol Phys* 1992; DOI: 10.1016/0360-3016(92)91025-I)

Patients treated with maximal safe resection and risk adapted chemotherapy ("8-in-1" + MTX). RT only to PF (54 Gy) and spine (36 Gy), excluding supratentorium. Trial closed early due to early neuroaxis failures. 9/13 failures in supratentorium. Supratentorial RT is necessary.

### CCG 9892 (Packer, *J Clin Oncol* 1999; http://jco.ascopubs.org/content/17/7/2127.abstract)

Phase II study of standard-risk patients treated with 23.4 Gy CSI and PF boost to 55.8 Gy with concurrent vincristine. Followed by adjuvant cisplatin/CCNU/vincristine. Five-year progression-free survival (PFS) 79%, similar to historical controls of patients treated to 36 Gy.

### Baby POG I (Duffner, *Neuro-Oncol* 1999; http://www.ncbi.nlm.nih.gov/pmc/articles/PMC1920752/)

Phase II trial delaying RT in infants <3 years treated with maximal safe surgery ➔ chemotherapy until age three or disease progression ➔ RT. For GTR and M0 infants, RT = 24 Gy CSI + 50 Gy PF boost. Five-year overall survival (OS) 69%. Overall, GTR 38%, OS 40%. No difference if RT delayed by 1 or 2 years.

### POG 8631/CCG 923 (Thomas, *J Clin Oncol* 2000; http://jco.ascopubs.org/content/18/16/3004.abstract)

Randomized standard-risk patients to 36 Gy CSI versus 23.4 Gy CSI followed by PF boost to 54 Gy (no chemo). Study closed prematurely due to high relapse in reduced CSI arm (5-year EFS: standard CSI 67% vs. reduced CSI 52%).

### CCG A9961 (Packer, *J Clin Oncol* 2006; DOI: 10.1200/JCO.2006.06.4980)

Randomized standard risk patients after 23.4 Gy CSI and 55.8 Gy PF boost with concurrent vincristine to two different chemotherapy regimens: (a) CCNU, cisplatin, and vincristine versus (b) cyclophosphamide, cisplatin, and vincristine. Five-year EFS 81%, OS 89%. No difference between chemo arms. Reduced dose CSI can be delivered with chemo safely excluding toxicities of higher dose CSI.

### COG ACNS0331 (Data not yet published)

Randomized standard risk patients to posterior fossa boost versus conformal tumor bed boost. Also randomized patients age three to seven to 18 Gy CSI versus 23.4 Gy CSI. All patients received same chemotherapy regimen. Awaiting study results.

# 46: NEUROBLASTOMA

*James Y. Rao, MD*
*Sahaja Acharya, MD*
*Stephanie M. Perkins, MD*

## WORKUP

### All Cases
- H&P
- CT or MRI primary, CT chest, abd, pelvis, MIBG scan
- Labs: CBC, CMP, UA, urinary VMA/HMA
- Bilateral bone marrow biopsy

### Considerations
- Most commonly arises in the adrenals
- Neuroblastoma (NB) patients have constitutional sx ("sick appearing")
- Tumors commonly have calcifications
- Skull and orbit bones are common sites of metastasis
- N-myc amp or DI = 1 associated with poorer prognosis
- Significant portion of infants have spontaneous regression

## TREATMENT RECOMMENDATIONS

### Based on COG Risk Groups
*Low Risk (as Defined in ANBL00B1)*
- Stage 1, Any
- Stage 2, N-myc not Amp, and Resection ≥50%
- Stage 4S, N-myc not Amp, DI >1, FH, and Asymp

*Intermediate Risk (as Defined in ANBL0531)*
- Stage 2, N-myc not Amp, and Bx/Resection <50%
- Stage 3 and Age <547 days
- Stage 3, Age ≥547 days, and FH
- Stage 4 and Age <365 days
- Stage 4, Age ≥365 days, DI >1, and FH
- Stage 4S, N-myc not Amp, and not low risk

*High Risk (as Defined in ANBL0532)*
- Stage 2, N-myc Amp
- Stage 3, N-myc Amp
- Stage 3, Age ≥547 days, N-myc not Amp, and UH
- Stage 4, N-myc Amp

- Stage 4, Age 365 to 546 days, and DI = 1
- Stage 4, Age 365 to 546 days, and UH
- Stage 4, Age ≥547 days
- Stage 4S, N-myc Amp

FH: favorable histology; UH: unfavorable histology; Amp: amplified; DI: DNA Index; Asymp: asymptomatic

| Low risk | Surgery, then observation<br>Observation after bx for stage 4S patients |
|---|---|
| Intermediate risk | Maximum safe resection<br>Chemotherapy based on biology<br>Second-look surgery considered for patients with initial unresectable disease or incomplete resection.<br>RT is controversial.<br>RT to residual or recurrent tumor not recommended in ANBL0531, which prefers additional chemo. |
| High risk | Induction chemotherapy<br>Surgical resection<br>Consolidation chemo/transplant<br>RT to primary site and to viable met<br>Maintenance cis-retinoic acid |
| Cord compression | Consider up-front chemo<br>RT or surgery for unresponsive disease |
| Symptomatic hepatomegaly | Whole liver radiation |
| Metastatic sites | Evaluate for MIBG positive met after induction chemotherapy. RT to be delivered after transplant. |

## TECHNICAL CONSIDERATIONS

### Simulation
- Simulate and treat with general anesthesia if necessary.
- Consider 4DCT for tumor locations in the thorax or upper abdomen susceptible to motion.

### Dose Prescription
- High Risk: 21.6 Gy in 1.8 Gy/fx if GTR and 36 Gy in 1.8 Gy/fx if gross residual (21.6 Gy + 14.4 Gy boost)
- Cord Compression: <3 years old: 9 Gy in 1.8 Gy/fx, ≥3 years old: 21.6 Gy in 1.8 Gy/fx

- Whole Liver Radiation: 4.5 Gy in 1.5 Gy/fx
- Metastasis: 21.6 Gy in 1.8 Gy/fx

## Target Delineation

*For High-Risk Disease*

- GTV1 = disease on imaging prior to surgery, + LN defined on path, corrected volumetrically after surgical resection but not at the point of attachment.
- GTV2 = volume of residual tumor after surgery and chemotherapy
- CTV1 = GTV1- + 1.5-cm anatomically confined expansion
- CTV2 = GTV2 + 1.0-cm anatomically confined expansion
- PTV1 = CTV1 + 0.5- to 1.0-cm expansion, this receives 21.6 Gy
- PTV2 = CTV2 + 0.5- to 1.0-cm expansion, this receives 14.4 Gy boost

For tumors located in the thorax or upper abdomen, an assessment should be made to determine the extent of motion. PTV margins should include motion as a component.

## Treatment Planning

- Conventional planning reasonable for lateralized tumors
- Consider 3D or intensity-modulated radiation therapy (IMRT) to reduce dose to normal structures

## FOLLOW UP

If asymptomatic: H&P with labs and catecholamines q3 months for 1 year, q6 months for 5 years, and afterward. Bone scan and MIBG at 3 months, then q6 months for 3 years.

## SELECTED STUDIES

### CCG 3891 (Matthay, *J Clin Oncol* 2009; DOI: 10.1200/JCO.2007.13.8925)

379 high-risk neuroblastoma patients treated induction chemotherapy and surgical resection, then randomized to myeloablative chemo, 10 Gy TBI, autologous bone marrow transplant versus intensive chemo. Patients then randomized to cis-RA versus no further therapy. Improved overall survival with ABMT/cis-RA 59% versus ABMT/no cis RA 41%, chemo/cis-RA 38%, and chemo/no cis-RA 36%.

### CCG 3891 RT Secondary Analysis (Haas-Kogan, *Int J Radiat Oncol Biol Phys* 2003)

For patients on CCG 3891, combined external beam radiation therapy (EBRT) 10 Gy to primary tumor site and addition of 10 Gy TBI resulted in improved local control of 52% compared to 10 Gy EBRT to primary tumor alone 22%. Suggests dose-response relationship for local RT.

### IMRT versus Conventional RT (Paulino, *Pediatr Blood Cancer* 2006)

IMRT reduced kidney doses for midline tumors. IMRT not superior to AP/PA fields for lateralized tumors.

# 47: WILMS' TUMOR

*James Y. Rao, MD*
*Sahaja Acharya, MD*
*Stephanie M. Perkins, MD*

## WORKUP

### All Cases

- H&P
- Abdominal US
- CT of chest and abdomen
- MRI brain and bone marrow biopsy for clear cell histology
- MRI brain for rhabdoid histology
- CBC, CMP, UA

### Considerations

- Tumor biopsy not recommended unless unresectable or bilateral
- Favorable histology (FH) includes patients without anaplastic, clear cell, or rhabdoid features.
- Stage III: "SLURP-Bx"—Spill, Lymph nodes, Unresectable, Rupture, Peritoneal disease, Piece meal resection, Positive margins, Biopsy

## TREATMENT RECOMMENDATIONS BY STAGE

Up-front surgical resection is routinely recommended in the United States. Up-front chemotherapy utilized in Europe.

RT recommendations depend on surgical findings and pathology.

| I–II FH | Surgery, chemotherapy<br>No radiation |
|---|---|
| III FH<br>I–III focal anaplasia<br>I–II diffuse anaplasia<br>I–III clear cell | Surgery, chemotherapy<br>Standard dose flank radiation |
| III diffuse anaplasia<br>I–III rhabdoid | Surgery, chemotherapy<br>High-dose flank radiation |
| Diffuse tumor spillage, tumor rupture, peritoneal seeding, or + cytology | Surgery, chemotherapy<br>Whole abdomen radiation |
| Metastatic disease | Manage abdominal disease as noted previously.<br>RT to lung, liver, brain, or bone metastasis |

## TECHNICAL CONSIDERATIONS

### Simulation

CT simulation with alpha cradle/vac lock bag. Arms up or akimbo to avoid flash coverage of arms. Consider 4DCT for whole lung RT, head extended for whole lung.

### Dose Prescription

- Standard dose flank radiation: 10.8 Gy in 1.8 Gy/fx
- High-dose flank radiation: 19.8 Gy in 1.8 Gy/fx (10.8 Gy in 1.8 Gy/fx in infants)
- Whole abdomen: 10.5 Gy in 1.5 Gy/fx, 21 Gy in 1.5 Gy/fx for diffuse anaplasia or rhabdoid histology, limit renal dose to 14.4 Gy with shielding (i.e., partial transmission PA block)
- Gross residual tumor after surgery: boost additional 10.8 Gy in 1.8 Gy/fx consider IMRT
- Whole lung: 12 Gy in 1.5 Gy/fx, 10.5 Gy 1.5 Gy fx, for <12 months old, 7.5 Gy in 1.5 Gy/fx, boost to residual disease after 2 weeks with conformal fields.
- Diffuse liver metastasis: 19.8 Gy in 1.8 Gy/fx to whole liver
- Brain metastasis: WBRT 21.6 Gy in 1.8 Gy/fx, then 10.8 Gy in 1.8 Gy/fx conformal boost
- Bone metastasis: 25.2 Gy in 1.8 Gy/fx (age <16 years)
- Unresected lymph nodes: 19.8 Gy in 1.8 Gy/fx
- Patients >16 years old may receive a higher total dose of 30.6 in 1.8 Gy/fx for brain mets, bone mets, or unresected nodes

### Target Delineation

- Flank: GTV = pre-op tumor and involved kidney, PTV = 1-cm expansion on GTV, medial border is past midline to 1 cm past contralateral vertebral body edge, other borders to include the PTV volume. Contour and include involved LN regions.
- Whole abdomen: Superior border is 1 cm above diaphragm, inferior border is bottom of obturator foramen, and lateral border is at least 1 cm beyond the abdominal wall. Block the femoral heads.
- Whole lung: Superior border is 1 cm above first rib, inferior border at L1. Include pleural recesses and block humeral heads. Consider IMRT.

### Treatment Planning
- AP/PA fields with 6-MV photons for flank, whole abdomen
- Consider IMRT for gross tumor boost, whole liver and whole lung
- RT is concurrent with chemo, start RT within 10 days of surgery

## FOLLOW UP

If asymptomatic: H&P q3 months for 3 years, then q6 months for 2 more years, then q2 years afterwards. CT chest, abdomen, pelvis at 3, 6, 12, and 18 months. CXR and abd US at other visits. No additional imaging after 5 years. See follow up schedules of AREN studies.

## SELECTED STUDIES

**NWTS-2 (D'Angio, *Cancer* 1981; DOI: 10.1002/1097-0142 (19810501)47:9<2302::AID-CNCR2820470933>3.0.CO;2-K)**
Stage I patients receiving chemo doublet do not require RT.

**NWTS-3 (D'Angio, *Cancer* 1989; DOI: 10.1002/1097-0142 (19890715)64:2<349::AID-CNCR2820640202>3.0.CO;2-Q)**
Stage II FH patients receiving chemo doublet do not require RT. Stage III FH patients can receive 10 Gy with chemo doublet.

**UKW-3 (Mitchell, *Eur J Cancer* 2006: DOI: 10.1016/j.ejca.2006.05.026)**
205 patients randomized to immediate surgery versus neoadjuvant chemo and delayed surgery. Patients received post-op therapy based on stage and histology at the time of surgery. Equivalent 5-year EFS 80% and OS 89%. Neoadjuvant chemotherapy resulted in 20% fewer children receiving RT or doxorubicin.

# 48: RHABDOMYOSARCOMA

*James Y. Rao, MD*
*Sahaja Acharya, MD*
*Stephanie M. Perkins, MD*

## WORKUP

### All Cases

- H&P
- Labs (CBC, CMP, LDH)
- CT/MRI primary, biopsy of primary site, bone marrow biopsy
- PET/CT
- For parameningeal head and neck sites: Brain MRI, CSF cytology, and neuroaxial imaging for + CSF

### Considerations

- Histology: Most favorable = embryonal (classic, spindle cell, and botyroid): most common in 2 to 6 years old. Less favorable = alveolar (most common in 15–19 years old), undifferentiated, anaplastic.
- Genes involved in alveolar: PAX3 or PAX7-FKHF fusions.
- Genetic syndromes associated with rhabdomyosarcoma: Beckwith-Widemann syndrome, Li Faumeni, and NF-1.
- Favorable organ sites: orbit, non-parameningeal head and neck, non-prostate/bladder genitourinary, and biliary.
- Parameningeal head and neck sites: middle ear, mastoid, nasal cavity, nasopharynx, infratemporal fossa, pterygopalatine fossa, paranasal sinus, and parapharyngeal space.
- Staging based on site (favorable vs. unfavorable) and TNM stage.

## CLINICAL GROUPING SYSTEM

| | |
|---|---|
| Ia | Confined to muscle of origin and completely resected |
| Ib | Contiguous extension beyond muscle of origin and completely resected |
| IIa | Microscopic residual disease and node negative |
| IIb | Regional nodal involvement without microscopic residual disease |

*(continued)*

| IIc | Regional nodal involvement and microscopic residual disease |
| IIIa | Gross residual disease after biopsy |
| IIIb | Gross residual disease after major resection |
| IV | Distant metastatic disease |

## TREATMENT RECOMMENDATIONS

General treatment paradigm is maximal safe resection with functional preservation followed by adjuvant therapy based on Group and histology as shown:

| | |
|---|---|
| Low-risk disease:<br>Embryonal histology only Stage 1–3, Groups I–II<br>Group III orbit<br>Stage 1, Group III, non-orbit | Vincristine/actinomycin D/cyclophosphamide (VAC)<br>No RT for Group I<br>RT for all other groups<br>Radiation at week 13 unless threat to vision/other functions |
| Intermediate-risk disease:<br>Embryonal histology Stage 2/3, Group III, non-orbit<br>Alveolar histology Stage 1–3, Groups I–III | Vincristine/actinomycin D/cyclophosphamide / vincristine/irinotecan + RT<br>RT at week 4 unless threat to vision/other functions |
| High-risk disease:<br>Any histology, Group IV, Stage IV | Vincristine/ doxorubicin/cyclophosphamide (VDC)/ifosphamide/etoposide(IE) + RT |

## TECHNICAL CONSIDERATIONS

### Simulation
Simulation is dependent on the location of primary site. Fuse pre- and post-op CT/MRI and/or PET/CT to aid treatment planning.

### Dose Prescription
- Group I: No RT for favorable histology, 36 Gy in 1.8 Gy/fx for unfavorable histology
- Group IIA: 36 Gy in 1.8 Gy/fx
- Group IIB/C: 41.4 Gy in 1.8 Gy/fx
- Group III orbit: 45 Gy in 1.8 Gy/fx
- Group III: 50.4 Gy in 1.8 Gy/fx

### Target Delineation

- GTV1 = Disease prior to surgery/chemo, including enlarged/unresected lymph nodes, can modify GTV to account for return of normal anatomy after tumor response (for pushing tumors)
- CTV1 = GTV1 + 1 cm
- PTV1 = CTV + at least 0.5 cm
- Orbit: CTV does not extend outside the orbit, entire orbit does not require treatment.
- Lymph nodes: When lymph nodes are involved in the entire lymph node chain should be treated.
- *volume reduction allowed after 36 Gy for rapidly responding tumors requiring 50.4 Gy (GTV2, CTV2 = GTV2 + 1 cm)

### Treatment Planning

- Organs at risk dependent on primary location
- IMRT or proton therapy for parameningeal sites

## FOLLOW UP

For the first year: Physical exam every 3 months (CBC, Platelets, chemistry panel, and blood pressure), CXR or chest CT every 3 months, Imaging of primary site every 3 months

Consider audiogram for parameningeal sites

## SELECTED STUDIES

### ARST0331 (Walterhouse et al., *J Clin Oncol* 2014; DOI: 10.1200/JCO.2014.55.6787)

Report on subset 1 of ARST0331: Stage 1/2, Group I/II or Stage 1 Group III orbit embryonal rhabdomyosarcoma, four cycles of VAC followed by four cycles of VA over 22 weeks, patients with Group II or III disease received radiation. Estimated 3-year FFS was 89%, overall survival rate was 98%. Concluded that shorter-duration therapy including lower-dose cyclophoshamide and RT did not compromise FFS with subset-one low-risk embryonal rhabdomyosarcoma.

### D9803 (Arndt CA et al., *J Clin Oncol* 2009; DOI: 10.1200/JCO.2009.22.3768)

Intermediate-risk rhabdomyosarcoma patients randomized to standard VAC versus VAC alternating with vincristine, topotecan, and cyclophosphamide (VAC/VTC). Four-year FFS was 73% with VAC and 68% with VAC/VTC ($P = .3$). No significant improvement with VAC/VTC.

**ARST0431 (Weigel BJ et al., *J Clin Oncol* 2015;**
**DOI: 10.1200/JCO.2015.63.4048)**
Patients with metastatic rhabdomyosarcoma received vincristine/
doxorubicin/cyclophosphamide, vincristine/irinotecan, and
etoposide/ifosfamide for a total of 54 weeks of therapy. Radiation
occurred at weeks 20 to 25 for primary site and weeks 47 to 52
for extensive metastatic disease. 199 patients enrolled. Three-
year EFS was 38%, 3-year OS was 56%. Toxicity similar to prior
rhabdomyosarcoma studies. Compared to historical cohort, there
was improvement in 3-year EFS for patients with one or no Oberlin
risk factors (3-year EFS 69%).

# 49: EWING'S SARCOMA

*James Y. Rao, MD*
*Sahaja Acharya, MD*
*Stephanie M. Perkins, MD*

## WORKUP

### All Cases

- H&P
- Labs: CBC, LFTs, LDH, and ESR
- X-ray of primary: "onion skinning," moth-eaten lesions in diaphysis
- CT and/or MRI, CT chest, bone scan ± PET
- Biopsy of primary and bone marrow biopsy

### Considerations

- Second most common bone cancer in children
- Male-to-female ratio (2:1), median age 14 years
- Most common presentation is in lower extremity/pelvis
- >90% of patients have t (11;22) or t (21;22) involving the EWS gene on chromosome 22.
- Negative prognostic factors: metastases, pelvic/truncal primary, proximal (vs. distal) primary, large tumors (>8 cm), age >17 years, high LDH, high ESR, poor response to induction chemotherapy, and no surgery.

## TREATMENT RECOMMENDATIONS

| Localized disease | Induction chemotherapy* → local therapy at 12 weeks (surgery ± RT) → consolidative chemotherapy* *vincristine, doxorubicin, cyclophosphamide alternating with etoposide and ifosfamide |
| --- | --- |
| Primary disseminated multifocal disease | Induction chemotherapy** → local therapy at 18 weeks (surgery ± RT) → chemotherapy ± stem cell transplant ** vincristine, doxorubicin, cyclophosphamide alternating with etoposide and ifosfamide |

## TECHNICAL CONSIDERATIONS

### Simulation

Simulation is dependent on location of primary site. Fuse pre- and post-op CT/MRI and/or PET/CT to aid treatment planning.

### Dose Prescription

Dose prescriptions to: (1) pre-chemotherapy and (2) post-chemotherapy volumes may differ.

- *A. Definitive radiation*:
  - PTV1: 45 Gy, PTV2: 55.8 Gy in 1.8 Gy/fx
- *B. Definitive radiation to vertebral body lesion*:
  - PTV1: 45 Gy, PTV2: 50.4 Gy in 1.8 Gy/fx
- *C. Post-op RT—microscopic residual*:
  - PTV1: 45 Gy, PTV2: 50.4 Gy in 1.8 Gy/fx
- *D. Post-op RT—gross residual*:
  - PTV1: 45 Gy, PTV2: 55.8 Gy in 1.8 Gy/fx
- *E. Special situations*:
  - *LN positive—resected*: PTV1: 50.4 Gy in 1.8 Gy/fx
  - *LN positive—unresected*: PTV1: 45 Gy, PTV2: 55.8 Gy in 1.8 Gy/fx
  - *Malignant ascites/diffuse peritoneal involvement*: Whole abdomen RT: 25 Gy in 1.5 Gy/ fx
  - *Lung metastases*: Whole lung RT: 15 Gy in 1.5 Gy/fx (if <6 years, then 12 Gy in 1.5 Gy/fx)
  - *Chest wall tumor/pleural nodules*: Chest wall tumor: PTV1: 30.6 Gy, PTV2 36 Gy in 1.8 Gy/fx, Pleural nodule: PTV1: 21.6 Gy, PTV2: 36 Gy in 1.8 Gy/fx, Hemithorax RT 15 Gy in 1.5 Gy/fx

### Target Delineation

- Contour GTV1 using prechemotherapy disease as defined by physical exam, CT, MRI, PET/CT (exclude pushing borders into body cavities)
- CTV1 = GV1 + 1 cm
- PTV1 = CTV + 0.5 cm
- Contour GTV2 using postchemotherapy disease as defined by physical exam, CT, MRI, PET/CT (exclude pushing borders into body cavities)
- CTV1 = GV1 + 1 cm

- PTV1 = CTV + 0.5 cm
- Refer to AEWS1031 for further contouring guidelines.

### Treatment Planning
- For extremity primaries, keep a strip of 1- to 2-cm skin <20 to 30 Gy to prevent lymphedema
- Dose >20 Gy can prematurely close epiphysis
- Organs at risk dependent on primary location

### FOLLOW UP

If asymptomatic: H&P with chest x-ray and x-ray of primary (± MRI) every 3 months for 2 years. After 2 years, can follow up with longer intervals.

Regular exams to monitor treatment sequelae: abnormal bone growth, weakening of bone (highest risk for fracture <18 months from completion of RT), lymphedema, and decreased range of motion of joint. Be cognizant of secondary malignancies.

### SELECTED STUDIES

#### INT-0091/IESS-III (Grier et al., *N Engl J Med* 2003; DOI: 10.1056/NEJMoa020890)
Randomized patients with Ewing's sarcoma, PNET of bone or primitive sarcoma of bone to vincristine-doxorubicin-cyclophosphamide (VDC) alone versus VDC alternating with ifosfamide and etoposide (IE). Twenty-three percent had metastatic disease. VDC/IE arm had significant improvement in OS (72% vs. 61%) and EFS (63% vs. 54%) in patients with nonmetastatic disease.

#### INT-0154 (Granowetter et al., *J Clin Oncol* 2009; DOI: 10.1200/JCO.2008.19.1478)
Randomized patients with non-metastatic Ewing's sarcoma of the bone or soft tissue to standard dose VDC/IE over 48 weeks or a dose intensified VDC/IE over 30 weeks. No OS or EFS benefit of dose escalation.

### COG AEWS0031 (Womer et al., *J Clin Oncol* 2012; DOI: 10.1200/JCO.2011.41.5703)

Patients with localized extradural Ewing's sarcoma were randomized to standard VDC/IE (q3 weeks) versus intensified VDC/IE (q2 weeks). Intensified arms had significant improvement in EFS (73% vs. 65%).

### Haeusler et al., *Cancer* 2010; DOI: 10.1002/cncr.24740

Secondary analysis of EURO-EWING 99 to determine the value of local treatment in patients with primary, disseminated multifocal Ewing's sarcoma. On multivariate analysis, absence of local therapy (surgery and/or RT) was a major risk factor (HR: 2.21, $P = .021$). Three-year EFS was 39% in patients who underwent local therapy of primary tumor and metastases vs. 14% in patients who did not undergo any local therapy ($P < .001$).

# 50: LEUKEMIA

*James Y. Rao, MD*
*Sahaja Acharya, MD*
*Stephanie M. Perkins, MD*


## WORKUP

### All Cases

- H&P
- Neuroimaging if symptomatic
- CBC, CMP, CSF, bone marrow biopsy, cytogenetics

### Considerations

Acute lymphoblastic leukemia (ALL) and acute myeloid leukemia (AML) are most common leukemias in children.

In general, treatment consists of induction, consolidation, delayed intensification, and maintenance phases of chemotherapy.

Classification of bone marrow involvement

- M1: <5% lymphoblasts
- M2: 5% to 25% lymphoblasts
- M3: >25% lymphoblasts

Classification of central nervous system involvement

- CNS1—negative cytology
- CNS2—positive cytology <5 WBC/mcL
- CNS3—positive cytology ≥5 WBC/mcL

Classification of treatment response to induction

Rapid early responder (RER)—M1 marrow on day 8 or 15 and M1 marrow with negative minimal residual disease (MRD) status on day 29.

Slow early responder (SER)—M2 or M3 marrow on day 15 or positive MRD status on day 29.

CNS and testicles considered sanctuary sites

In ALL, recent trials have preserved RT for CNS prophylaxis in certain risk groups, CNS3 disease, T-cell ALL, or recurrence.

In AML, recent trials in North America have largely eliminated cranial RT. AML02 did not use RT even for CNS3 patients. In recurrent AML, intrathecal and systemic chemotherapy are used. Bone marrow failure often rapidly follows apparent isolated CNS failure in AML. Palliative RT useful for chloromas.

Total body irradiation (TBI) is used as part of conditioning regimens prior to stem cell transplant and may be myeloablative or nonmyeloablative.

## TREATMENT RECOMMENDATIONS

*For ALL, risk categories as defined in AALL0331*

- Standard risk: B-precursor, WBC <50k, age 1 to 10 years
- High risk: all others not in standard or very high-risk groups
- Very high risk: Ph+, t(9;22)(q34;q11), hypodiploid clone, induction failure, or mixed-lineage leukemia (MLL) rearrangement with SER after induction.
- T-cell ALL: It has separate classification system. See AALL0434.

All patients will typically receive systemic and intrathecal chemotherapy, the following table includes only the radiation therapy recommendations.

| | |
|---|---|
| When recommended, cranial RT is typically given during delayed intensification or at the start of maintenance chemotherapy depending on study protocol or institutional practice. ALL with CNS3—any risk category | Therapeutic cranial RT |
| Standard risk ALL—CNS1 or CNS2 | No prophylactic cranial radiation |
| High-risk ALL—all slow early responder patients, patients with MLL rearrangements, patients pretreated with steroids | Prophylactic cranial RT |
| High-risk ALL—CNS1 or CNS2 and not meeting the preceding criteria | No prophylactic cranial radiation |
| Very high risk ALL—CNS1 or CNS2 | Prophylactic cranial RT |
| T-cell ALL—Intermediate and high risk—CNS1/2 | Prophylactic cranial RT |
| CNS relapse | Early relapse: craniospinal radiation<br>Late (≥18 months): cranial RT only |
| Testicular involvement or relapse | Bilateral testicular radiation if disease persistent at the end of induction or reinduction chemotherapy |

(*continued*)

| Ocular involvement or relapse | If anterior chamber: electron beam RT<br>If retina or choroid: consider as CNS failure. Local eye and optic nerve RT or cranial RT with eye boost |
|---|---|
| Symptomatic chloroma | Involved site radiation |
| Transplant conditioning | Myeloablative TBI may be used for ALL and AML patients requiring transplant such as those with very high risk or recurrence.<br>Nonmyeloablative TBI is occasionally used in patients with poor performance status but its role is not well established in pediatric patients |

## TECHNICAL CONSIDERATIONS

### Simulation

- Simulate with aquaplast mask and anesthesia if necessary.
- If craniospinal, sim with head extended. Prone or supine positioning is appropriate for CSI depending on institutional practice.
- TBI setup varies by institutional practice. At Washington University, adolescents and adults are treated with opposed lateral beams in a seated position. Infants are treated AP/PA using supine/prone positioning and lung blocking. Scatter screen in beam path.

### Dose Prescription

- Prophylactic cranial RT: 12 Gy in 1.5 Gy/fx
- Therapeutic cranial RT: 18 Gy in 1.8 Gy/fx
- CNS relapse: Short remission (<18 months) 24 Gy to whole brain and 15 Gy to spine in 1.5 Gy/fx, long remission (≥18 months) 18 Gy to whole brain in 1.5 Gy/fx. Dose may be reduced to 15 Gy if there has been prior cranial radiation to >20 Gy
- Testicular RT: 24 Gy in 2 Gy/fx
- Anterior chamber of eye: 12 Gy in 2 Gy/fx en-face electrons
- Retina or choroid involvement: 24 Gy in 12/Gy fx to eye, consider cranial RT as posterior recurrence considered CNS failure

- Chloroma: 24 Gy in 2 Gy/fx
- Myeloablative TBI: 12 to 14.4 Gy in 2 to 2.2 Gy/fx BID at low-dose rate <10 to 12 cGy/min
- Nonmyeloablative TBI: 2 to 4 Gy in single fraction at low-dose rate

In patients receiving cranial RT and planned to receive TBI, subtract the TBI dose from the planned cranial RT dose. Example: For a very high-risk patient with CNS3 disease planned for 12-Gy TBI in preparation for transplant, 6 Gy in 3 fx just prior to TBI is adequate for a patient who otherwise would have receive 18-Gy cranial dose.

**Target Delineation**
- Cranial radiation: Include the entire brain and meninges including the posterior halves of the globes of the eyes and cribriform plate. Caudal border below the skull at C2 level.
- Craniospinal radiation: Cranial fields as noted previously and match to spine field. Caudal border of cranial field located above shoulders. Avoid divergence through the mouth. Contour thecal sac to define inferior borders of spine field. Lateral borders of spine field should cover entire vertebral body with 1-cm margin. Dose to cover the entire vertebral body anteriorly. Junction shifts cranially 1 cm every 5 fractions.
- TBI: Prescription point is to midline. Monitor units and compensator calcs based on clinical setup, patient hip, and lateral head measurements.

**Treatment Planning**
- For cranial or CSI, 6-MV photons and conventional or 3D planning.
- For TBI at Washington University, 6-MV photons with right/left lateral fields at 300-cm source to axis distance, low dose rate, scatter screen, and head compensator is used for adolescents and adults. AP/PA beams, scatter screen, and lung compensators are used for infants.

**FOLLOW UP**

If asymptomatic: H&P with labs weekly during induction, start of consolidation and delayed intensification, q4 weeks in maintenance.

## SELECTED STUDIES

### St. Jude's Total Therapy XV (Pui, *N Engl J Med* 2009; DOI: 10.1056/NEJMoa0900386)

498 patients with ALL were treated with chemo and intrathecal prophylaxis without CSI. Five-year EFS and OS were 85.6% and 93.5%, respectively. Five-year risk of any CNS relapse was 3.9%. CNS3 or a traumatic lumbar puncture with blast cells and a high level of minimal residual disease (≥1%) after induction associated with poorer EFS. Risk factors for CNS relapse included t(1;19) (TCF3-PBX1), any CNS involvement at diagnosis, and T-cell ALL.

### POG 9412 (Barredo, *J Clin Oncol* 2006; DOI: 10.1200/JCO.2005.03.3373)

76 patients with first CNS relapse of ALL treated with systemic and intrathecal chemotherapy for 12 months and then 24-Gy cranial/15-Gy spinal RT if <18-month remission or 18-Gy cranial radiation if ≥18-month remission. 97.4% achieved second remission. Four-year EFS for patients with early or late relapse were 51.6% and 77.7%.

### St. Jude's Testicular RT (Hijiya, *Leukemia* 2005; DOI: 10.4103/0019-509X.63002)

Isolated testicular relapse very rare due to HD-MTX. Testicle RT is unnecessary if responsive to chemo. In 811 patients on St. Jude's trials, 19 (2.3%) had testicular disease at diagnosis. Two patients received testicular RT due to residual disease after induction. Both subsequently died due to bone marrow relapse.

### UK MRC Ocular RT (Somervaille, *Br J Haematol* 2003; DOI: 10.1046/j.1365-2141.2003.04280.x)

20 cases of ocular relapse represented 2.2% of ALL relapses in UK MRC studies. All 11 children who received CNS relapse protocol chemo and RT have survived. Seven of 11 survivors received cranial, craniospinal, or TBI in addition to ocular RT. Used ocular doses of 8 to 24 Gy. Recommend dose >20 Gy.

### MSKCC Chloroma (Bakst, *Int J Radiat Oncol Biol Phys* 2012; DOI: 10.1016/j.ijrobp.2011.02.057)

Recommend treating symptomatic chloromas to at least 20 Gy, and propose 24 Gy in 12 fractions as appropriate regimen.

# 51: PALLIATIVE RADIATION

*James B. Yu, MD, MHS*

## WORKUP

### All Cases

- H&P (including performance status)
- There should be pathologic confirmation of cancer, and ideally pathologic confirmation of cancer metastases. If no pathologic evidence of cancer metastases, proceed with great caution.
- Tumors targeted for radiation require both radiologic evidence of tumor and clinical correlation with pain.

## TREATMENT RECOMMENDATIONS BY TYPE OF PALLIATION

| | |
|---|---|
| Bone metastases (non-vertebral) | Use 8 Gy in 1 fx if survival limited. Do not use more than 10 fractions. |
| Bone metastases (vertebral) 1–3 metastases, no cord compression | If single and solitary, strongly consider radiosurgery. If no more than 3 sites, good performance status and expected prolonged survival, can consider radiosurgery. |
| Bone metastases (vertebral) multiple metastases, no cord compression | Consider at least 20 Gy in 5 fx or longer fractionation (30 Gy in 10 fx) given the potential morbidity of recurrence. Consider single fraction in patients with very short life expectancy (<6 months) |
| Bone metastases (vertebral), with cord compression— Surgical candidate | Surgical decompression and post-op radiation shown to improve days of walking compared to radiation alone. |
| Bone metastases (vertebral), with cord compression— Non-surgical candidate | 30 Gy in 10 fx preferred if survival limited. If aggressive therapy desired, can consider radiosurgery. |
| Retreatment of boney metastases | Retreatment can be safely performed in most cases |
| Bleeding (unresectable gastric) | 30 Gy in 10 fx can be considered |
| Bleeding (unresectable colorectal) | 25 Gy in 5fx can be considered |

(continued)

*(continued)*

| Bleeding (bladder) | 21 Gy in 3fx equivalent to 35 Gy in 10 fx. Could also consider 20 Gy in 5 fx, or 30 Gy in 10 fx |
| Bleeding (Gyn) | 3.7 Gy/fx × 4 fx over 2 days (BID treatment) can be considered. 30 Gy in 10 fx can be considered |

## TECHNICAL CONSIDERATIONS

### Simulation

■ Simulate with patient comfort in mind. Be aware of limited mobility or range of motion.

### *For Spine Radiosurgery*

■ Careful immobilization is required. Simulate supine, ideally with full body immobilization (such as body-fix bag). For cervical or upper thoracic vertebral tumors, use a head and shoulders mask. Image guidance is necessary, and preferably a delivery system that allows 6 degrees of freedom in patient alignment (with robotic treatment table or robotic linear accelerator). For visualization of the spinal cord and canal, MRI or CT myelogram is required—ideally obtained with patient in treatment position.

### Dose Prescription

■ Consider single fraction treatment if at all possible, in particular for patients with life expectancy shorter than 6 months.
■ Limit palliative courses to 10 fractions at most. Acceptable fractionation schema includes 30 Gy in 10 fx, 24 Gy in 6 fx, 20 Gy in 5 fx, and 8 Gy in 1 fx.

### *For Spine Radiosurgery*

■ A prescription dose of 16 Gy is adequate, though some institutions use higher doses. With higher doses, monitor for potential vertebral body compression fracture posttreatment, particularly those with high Spine Instability Neoplastic Score (SINS).

### Target Delineation

■ For standard palliative radiation, though target delineation should ideally encompass the entire tumor, if the field of treatment is anticipated to cause undue toxicity, fields can be reduced as needed. For standard vertebral body radiotherapy, include one additional vertebral body above and below involved vertebrae.

*For Spine Radiosurgery*

- Ideally adhere to RTOG 0631 guidelines. Clinical tumor volume (CTV) should take into account involvement of the body, pedicles, and dorsal elements of the vertebrae. When possible (e.g., if only the body or dorsal elements are involved) avoid a circumferential CTV. CTV to PTV expansion will depend on the institution's ability to immobilize and track movement. Typically expansion is 1 to 3 mm.

## Planning

- For standard palliative radiation, use intensity-modulated radiation therapy (IMRT) and image guidance sparingly.

*For Spine Radiosurgery*

- Spinal cord volume can be defined at the level of the target vertebrae, with an additional 6 mm cranial and caudad. Max spinal cord point dose should be 14 Gy, with a maximum of 10% of the cord volume receiving >10 Gy.

## Other Considerations

- Get palliative care involved early for all patients with metastatic disease.

*For Spine Radiosurgery*

- Pain flare postspine SRS usually 1 day can be up to 5 days postradiation. For patients undergoing spine radiosurgery, therefore consider a brief course of low/moderate dose corticosteroid therapy (such as dexamethasone 4 mg PO QD) × 2 to 3 days, immediately following treatment.
- *Be aware that palliative care encompasses not only treatment of pain and physical discomfort, but also depression, anxiety, and psychosocial issues. Consider engagement with your palliative care team or social work team.*

## FOLLOW UP

Follow up 1 month posttreatment unless transport is difficult for the patient.

## SELECTED STUDIES

### Patchell Cord Compression Trial (Patchell, *Lancet* 2005; DOI:10.1016/S0140-6736(05)66954-1)

Surgical decompression plus post-op radiation superior to radiation alone. Surgery + radiation therapy (RT) had median 122 days walking versus RT alone (13 days median). Lower need for corticosteroids and opioids with surgical group.

### Rades Multicenter (Rades, *Cancer* 2004; DOI: 10.1002/cncr.20633)

Prospective multicenter study compared 30 Gy in 10 fx to 40 Gy in 20 fx and found no differences. 30 Gy in 10 fx preferred given shorter length.

### ASTRO Consensus Guidelines for Palliative Thoracic Radiation in Lung Cancer (Rodriguez, *Pract Rad Onc* 2011; DOI: 10.1016/j.prro.2011.01.005)

30 Gy in 10 fx, or fewer fractions, are preferred for palliation of thoracic symptoms.

### NEJM Palliative Care Study (Temel, *N Engl J Med* 2010; DOI: 10.1056/NEJMoa1000678)

Early involvement of palliative care improves survival and quality of life, and reduces unnecessary chemotherapy administration.

### RTOG 97-14 (Hartsell, *J Natl Cancer Inst* 2013; DOI: 10.1093/jnci/dji139)

8 Gy in 1 fx arm had higher retreatment rate than 30 Gy in 10 fx arm for painful bone metastases. However, patients who underwent 8 Gy had the same rate of pain relief as those who underwent 30 Gy. Complete and partial response of pain was 15 to 18% and 48 to 50%, respectively. 8 Gy better tolerated.

### Phase 1-2 SBRT for Spine Metastases (Wang, *Lancet Oncol* 2012; DOI: 10.1016/S1470-2045(11)70384-9)

This study investigated 146 patients with 166 non-cord-compressing spine metastases. Complete response (by brief pain inventory) was 54% at 6 months after stereotactic body radiation therapy (SBRT). Progression-free survival after SBRT 72.4%. SBRT well tolerated for mechanically stable spinal metastases.

### Ryu Cord Compression SRS Trial (Ryu, *Cancer* 2010; DOI: 10.1002/cncr.24993)

Prospective Phase II trial found radiosurgical decompression of metastatic epidural cord compression possible and associated with neurological improvement. SRS resulted in an approximately 70% reduction in volume of epidural tumors, with 84% neuropreservation.

### RTOG 0631 - Phase 2/3 of IG-SRS for 1-3 Metastases (Ryu, *PRO* 2014; DOI: 10.1016/j.prro.2013.05.001)

16 Gy single fraction SRS delivered for 1 to 3 spine metastases. Compliance to protocol among 65 institutions was excellent. Hopefully results of the randomized comparison of 16 Gy SRS versus 8 Gy (conventionally delivered) will be reported soon.

### SINS Score (Sahgal, *J Clin Oncol* 2013; DOI: 10.1200/JCO.2013.50.1411)

Lytic tumor, baseline spinal misalignment, and vertebral body collapse pre-radiosurgery are all risk factors for vertebral body compression fracture postradiosurgery, in particular with higher doses of treatment (>18 Gy). Consider pre-radiosurgical stabilization if these factors exist.

# APPENDIX 1: RADIATION THERAPY SYMPTOM MANAGEMENT

*Aida Amado, ACNP-BC*

- Skin
  - General measures
    - Gently wash skin with lukewarm water and mild soap
    - Apply unscented, lanolin-free moisturizer 2 to 3 times daily
    - Avoid irritants, sun exposure, alcohol-based topical gels, and extreme temperatures
    - Wear loose fitting clothes
  - Pruritus
    - Topical corticosteroids with low- to mid-potency for example, triamcinolone or mometasone
  - Erythema, dry desquamation—early radiation dermatitis
    - Hydrophilic moisturizers
  - Moist desquamation
    - Wound dressings: nonadherent, hydrogel, or hydrocolloid dressings
    - Pain management as needed
    - Observe for secondary infection, candidiasis
  - Ulceration
    - Possible discontinuation of radiotherapy, referral to wound specialists, possible surgical referral for debridement
    - Pain management as needed
- Nervous system
  - General measures
    - Tumor-related edema—glucocorticoids.
    - In symptomatic patients start 24 to 48 prior to radiotherapy
    - In asymptomatic patients consider prophylaxis or observation
    - Degree of edema and clinical symptoms to guide dosing
      - Nausea, vomiting, vertigo, cognitive dysfunction, visual changes, generalized weakness, focal neurological changes, headache
    - Taper according to clinical symptoms
  - Seizures
    - Assess for other metabolic causes, progression of disease, cerebrovascular accident, or paraneoplastic syndromes

- Start anti-convulsive medication
- No documented role for prophylactic anti-convulsive

■ Eyes
  ■ General measures
    - Manage dry, irritated eyes, and inflammation
  ■ Eye irritation
    - Artificial tears: drops or gel formulations: over the counter natural tears, Lacri Lube
    - Topical analgesic: for example, Proparacaine hydrochloride 5% 2 gtss BID
    - Antibiotic + anti-inflammatory preparation for example, Tobradex (tobramycin + dexamethasone)
    - Observe for secondary infection

■ Nose/sinuses
  ■ General measures
    - Manage dry, irritated nasal passages, and inflammation
  ■ Nasal mucositis/sinusitis
    - Dry/painful nasal passages-saline sprays, topical analgesics for example, ocean spray, lidocaine gel
    - Anti-histamine therapy as needed to decrease drainage
    - Antibiotic therapy if infection is suspected

■ Ear
  ■ Otitis media
    - Antibiotic therapy for example, amoxicillin
  ■ NSAIDs or other pain management as needed
    Radiotherapy-induced eustachian tube edema
    - Start with a decongestant
    - Short course of steroids if no improvement with decongestant
  ■ Radiotherapy-induced otitis externa
    - Hydrocortisone otic
    - NSAIDs
    - Topical analgesic
    - Consider neomycin/polymixin/hydrocortisone otic if suspected bacterial infection

■ Oral cavity
  ■ General measures
    - Encourage good oral hygiene, warm baking soda rinses, daily brushing with mild toothbrush, fluoride use, decreased use of oral irritants/spicy foods

- Mucositis
  - Baking soda rinses
  - Topical anesthetic rinses with lidocaine base: swish and swallow
  - Will require oral analgesics; opiate therapy plus adjuvants, that is, gabapentin
  - Assess for HSV and candidiasis
- Oral candidiasis
  - Nystatin oral suspension, fluconazole, or Mycelex troche for refractory candidiasis
- Ulceration
  - Pain management with opioid therapy
- Infection
  - Antibiotic therapy
- Thick, ropy secretions
  - Consider guaifenesin, scopalamine
  - Consider home suction
  - Increase oral hydration
- Dysgeusia
  - Pharmacological strategies without evidence to prove effectiveness. Recommend dietary counseling
- Xerostomia
  - OTC artificial saliva or other OTC products to moisten oral cavity, baking soda rinse
  - Dietary counseling
  - Consider medication: that is pilocarpine, cevimeline
  - Counsel patient on oral hygiene, fluoride protection for nonedentulous patients
  - Humidifier, acupuncture
- Trismus
  - Passive range of motion exercise; refer to speech and/or physical therapy
- Decreased nutritional intake
  - Consider feeding tube if patient unable to maintain adequate nutritional needs, hydration status
- Neck/throat
  - Esophagitis
    - Will require oral analgesics; opiate therapy
    - Topical anesthetic with lidocaine base; swish/swallow
    - Consider oral antifungal, fluconazole, for possible candidiasis
  - Fibrosis
    - Neck exercises; physical therapy referral

- Thyroiditis
  - Post-treatment—monitor TSH, manage abnormal values with thyroid hormones or refer to primary care doctor/endocrinology
- Lymphedema
  - Lymphedema referral 2 to 3 weeks post-treatment
- Breast
  - Abscess/inflammation
    - Consider drainage, antibiotic therapy
  - Radiation fibrosis
    - Teach patient daily massage of breast
    - If severe, can consider pentoxifylline 400 mg TID + Vitamin E 1,000 IU daily
  - Lymphedema—referral to lymphedema clinic: manual lymph drainage, pressure wraps, education
- Thorax
  - Pneumonitis
    - Be cognizant of time frame
    - Acute pneumonitis can be seen 4 to 12 weeks following radiotherapy
    - Late pneumonitis develops 4 to 6 months after radiotherapy and can continue to progress
    - Glucocorticoids—start with at least 60 mg Prednisone daily × 2 weeks with slow taper over several months, as symptoms tolerate
  - Cough
    - Assess for pneumonia, pneumonitis, pulmonary fibrosis
    - Encourage incentive spirometer or deep breathing exercises
    - Cough suppressants, inhaled corticosteroids, oral steroids
  - Pneumonia—treat accordingly including antibiotics
  - Pulmonary fibrosis—glucocorticoid, consider pentoxifylline 400 mg TID + Vitamin E 1,000 IU daily
    - Guaifenesin to assist with sputum expectoration
    - Encourage incentive spirometer or deep breathing exercises
- GI tract
  - GERD
    - H2 blocker or PPI
  - Esophagitis
    - Pain management

- Topical anesthetic with lidocaine base
- Consider empiric treatment of candidiasis
- Hiccups
  - Treat the cause when known
  - No high-level evidence for pharmacologic therapy, but baclofen, gabapentin, metoclopramide, and chlorpromazine, haloperidol effective in cases
- Motility issues
  - Metoclopramide if not contraindicated
  - Bowel regimen for constipation if patient on opiate therapy
  - Dietary counseling
- Nausea/vomiting
  - Consensus recommendation is serotonin 5-HT3 receptor antagonist, with or without dexamethasone
  - For radiation to upper abdomen or TBI, recommend premedication with anti-emetic daily prior to radiotherapy
  - Assess history of gastritis, treat accordingly starting with H2 blocker progressing to PPI as needed
  - Assess bowel status
- Diarrhea
  - Start with over the counter anti-diarrheal, such as, Imodium. Progress to prescription anti-diarrheal if no relief from over the counter medications
  - Assess dietary intake of fiber, fluids
- Acute proctitis
  - May occur during or within 6 weeks of radiotherapy completion
  - Assess for other underlying gastrointestinal issues such as *Clostridium difficile*, ulcerative colitis, diverticulitis
  - Manage with antidiarrheal medications and hydration
  - On rare occasions, patient may need a small treatment break
  - Counsel patient on skin care secondary to frequent stools
  - Consider low-residue diet
- Chronic proctitis
  - Mild symptoms may not warrant any intervention
  - Severe symptoms; recommend sucralfate or glucocorticoid enemas
  - Consider low-residue diet, gastrointestinal referral

- Genitourinary/gynecological
  - Cystitis
    - Obtain urinalysis, assess for infection
    - NSAIDs for bladder pain
    - Dysuria—phenazopyridine; start with over the counter dose, increase to prescription dose as needed
    - Referral to urology if no improvement
  - Bladder spasms
    - Recommend antispasmodics or anticholinergics
  - Chronic radiation cystitis
    - Changes most likely will be permanent
    - Refer to urology
    - Hematuria
      - Sodium pentosan polysulfate has shown improvement in radiation-induced hematuria
  - Urethral edema
    - NSAIDs or glucocorticoids
  - Vaginal mucositis
    - Wash with mild soap, Sitz baths
    - Vaginal douches: diluted hydrogen peroxide/water
  - Vaginal stenosis
    - Estrogen creams, if not contraindicated, have been shown to improve dyspareunia
    - Vaginal dilators are commonly used
- Anxiety—treatment related
  - General measures
    - Educate patient on positioning, treatment devices
    - Assess claustrophobia
    - Prescribe low dose anxiolytic as premedication
- Pain management
  - General measures
    - Goal is to provide optimal pain relief with minimal adverse effects
    - Begin with nonopioids, then mild opioids, then stronger opioids
    - For severe pain in adults, starting dose is morphine 30 mg daily or equivalent
    - Consider constipation prophylaxis

# APPENDIX 2: NORMAL TISSUE TOLERANCES

*Tomasz Bista, MS*

## TABLE A2.1: TISSUE TOLERANCES FRACTIONATED

| Organ | Type | Conventional Volume/Dose |
|---|---|---|
| Bladder | Vol (%) | <15% above 80 Gy; <25% above 75 Gy; <35% above 70 Gy; <50% above 65 Gy |
| Bone: Fem. Heads | Max dose | <54 Gy |
| Bone: Fem. Heads | Vol (%) | <10% above 50 Gy; <50% above 45 Gy |
| Bone: Mandible | Max dose | <72 Gy |
| Bone: Mandible | Vol (mL) | <1 mL above 70 Gy |
| Bowel: Duodenum | Vol (mL) | <5 mL above 56 Gy; <30 mL above 45 Gy |
| Bowel: Rectum | Vol (%) | <15% above 75 Gy; <20% above 70 Gy; <25% above 65 Gy; <35% above 60 Gy; <50% above 50 Gy |
| Bowel: Small intestine | Max dose | <54 Gy |
| Bowel: Small intestine | Vol (mL) | <10 mL above 50 Gy; <135 mL above 45 Gy |
| Bowel: Stomach | Max dose | <54 Gy |
| Bowel: Stomach | Vol (%) | <2% above 50 Gy; <25% above 45 Gy |
| Brachial Plexus | Max dose | <66 Gy |
| Brachial Plexus | Vol (%) | <5% above 60 Gy |
| Brain | Max dose | 60 Gy (<3% risk of necrosis): 72 Gy (5% risk of necrosis) |
| Brainstem | Tolerance dose | Entire brainstem <54 Gy |
| Brainstem | Vol (%) | <1 mL above 59 Gy |
| Brain: Pituitary | Mean dose | <40 Gy |
| Cauda Equina | Max dose | <60 Gy |
| Chiasm | Max dose | <55 Gy |
| Ears: Cochlea | Mean dose | <45 Gy (<35 Gy if pt treated with cisplatinum) |
| Ears: Cochlea | Vol (%) | <5% above 55 Gy |
| Esophagus | Mean dose | <34 Gy |

*(continued)*

## TABLE A2.1: TISSUE TOLERANCES FRACTIONATED (*CONTINUED*)

| Organ | Type | Conventional Volume/Dose |
|---|---|---|
| Esophagus | Vol (%) | <20% above 70 Gy; <40% above 50 Gy |
| Eyes: Lens | Max dose | <7 Gy |
| Eyes: Optic nerve | Max dose | <55 Gy |
| Eyes: Retina | Max dose | <50 Gy |
| Eyes: Retina | Mean dose | <35 Gy |
| Heart | Vol (%) | <46% above 30 Gy |
| Heart | Mean dose | <26 Gy |
| Kidneys: Bilateral | Mean dose | <18 Gy |
| Kidney: Bilateral | Vol(%) | <20% above 28 Gy; <30% above 23 Gy; <32% above 20 Gy; <55% above 12 Gy |
| Lacriminal gland | Max dose | <40 Gy |
| Lacriminal gland | Mean dose | <26 Gy |
| Larynx | Max dose | <66 Gy |
| Larynx | Mean dose | <44 Gy |
| Liver | Mean dose | <30 Gy |
| Liver | Vol (%) | <30% above 30 Gy; <50% above 20 Gy |
| Lungs | Mean dose | <20 Gy |
| Lungs | Vol (%) | <35% above 20 Gy, <45% above 10 Gy, <65% above 5 Gy |
| Ipsi lung (breast cancer cases) | Vol (%) | <10% above 25 Gy |
| Optic nerve | Max dose | <54 Gy |
| Oral cavity | Mean dose | <30 Gy |
| Parotid Glands: bilateral | Mean dose | <25 Gy |
| Parotid gland: One | Mean dose | <20 Gy |
| Penile bulb | Mean dose to 95% volume | <50 Gy |
| Pharyngeal constrictor | Mean dose | <50 Gy |
| Spinal cord | Max dose | <50 Gy |
| Submandibular gland | Mean dose | <35 Gy |

**TABLE A2.2: TISSUE TOLERANCES STEREOTACTIC**

| Organ | 1 Fraction | | 3 Fractions | | 5 Fractions | |
|---|---|---|---|---|---|---|
| | Type | Volume/Dose | Type | Volume/Dose | Type | Volume/Dose |
| Bladder wall | Max dose | <18.4 Gy | Max dose | <28 Gy | Max dose | <38 Gy |
| Bladder wall | Vol (mL) | <15 mL above 11.4 Gy | Vol (mL) | <15 mL above 16.8 Gy | Vol (mL) | <15 mL above 18.3 Gy |
| Bone: Fem. Heads | Vol (mL) | <10 mL above 14 Gy | Vol (mL) | <10 mL above 21.9 Gy | Vol (mL) | <10 mL above 30 Gy |
| Bone: Ribs | Max dose | <30 Gy | Max dose | <36.9 Gy | Max dose | <43 Gy |
| Bone: Ribs | Vol (mL) | <1 mL above 22 Gy | Vol (mL) | <1 mL above 28.8 Gy | Vol (mL) | <1 mL above 35 Gy |
| Bowel: Colon/Rectum | Max dose | <18.4 Gy | Max dose | <28.2 Gy | Max dose | <38 Gy |
| Bowel: Colon/Rectum | Vol (mL) | <20 mL above 14.3 Gy | Vol (mL) | <20 mL above 24 Gy | Vol (mL) | <20 mL above 25 Gy |
| Bowel: Duodenum | Max dose | <12.4 Gy | Max dose | <22.2 Gy | Max dose | <32 Gy |
| Bowel: Duodenum | Vol (mL) | <5 mL above 11.2 Gy | Vol (mL) | <5 mL above 16 Gy | Vol (mL) | <5 mL above 18 Gy |
| Bowel: Duodenum | Vol (mL) | <10 mL above 9 Gy | Vol (mL) | <10 mL above 11.4 Gy | Vol (mL) | <10 mL above 12.5 Gy |
| Bowel: Jejunum/Ileum | Max dose | <15.4 Gy | Max dose | <25.2 Gy | Max dose | <35 Gy |
| Bowel: Jejunum/Ileum | Vol (mL) | <5 mL above 11.5 Gy | Vol (mL) | <5 mL above 17.7 Gy | Vol (mL) | <5 mL above 19.5 Gy |

(continued)

# TABLE A2.2: TISSUE TOLERANCES STEREOTACTIC (CONTINUED)

| Organ | 1 Fraction | | 3 Fractions | | 5 Fractions | |
|---|---|---|---|---|---|---|
| | Type | Volume/Dose | Type | Volume/Dose | Type | Volume/Dose |
| Bowel: Stomach | Max dose | <12.4 Gy | Max dose | <22.2 Gy | Max dose | <32 Gy |
| Bowel: Stomach | Vol (mL) | <10 mL above 11 Gy | Vol (mL) | <10 mL above 16.5 Gy | Vol (mL) | <10 mL above 18 Gy |
| Brachial Plexus: Ipsilat | Max dose | <17.5 Gy | Max dose | <24 Gy | Max dose | <30.5 Gy |
| Brachial Plexus: Ipsilat | Vol (mL) | <3 mL above 14 Gy | Vol (mL) | <3 mL above 20.4 Gy | Vol (mL) | <3 mL above 27 Gy |
| Brain | Vol (mL) | <10 mL above 10 Gy | | | | |
| Brainstem | Max dose | <12.5 Gy | Max dose | <23.1 Gy | Max dose | <31 Gy |
| Brainstem | Vol (mL) | <0.5 mL above 10 Gy | Vol (mL) | <0.5 mL above 18 Gy | Vol (mL) | <0.5 mL above 23 Gy |
| Bronchus (small) | Max dose | <13.3 Gy | Max dose | <23.1 Gy | Max dose | <33 Gy |
| Bronchus (small) | Vol (mL) | 0.5 mL above 12.4 Gy | Vol (mL) | <0.5 mL above 18.9 Gy | Vol (mL) | <0.5 mL 21 Gy |
| Bronchus/Trachea | Max dose | <20.2 Gy | Max dose | <30 Gy | Max dose | <40 Gy |
| Bronchus/Trachea | Vol (mL) | <4 mL above 10.5 Gy | Vol (mL) | <4 mL above 15 Gy | Vol (mL) | <4 mL above 16.5 Gy |
| Cauda equina | Max dose | <16 Gy | Max dose | <24 Gy | Max dose | <32 Gy |
| Cauda equina | Vol (mL) | <5 mL above 14 Gy | Vol (mL) | <5 mL above 21.9 Gy | Vol (mL) | <5 mL above 30 Gy |

*(continued)*

# TABLE A2.2: TISSUE TOLERANCES STEREOTACTIC (CONTINUED)

| Organ | 1 Fraction | | 3 Fractions | | 5 Fractions | |
|---|---|---|---|---|---|---|
| | Type | Volume/Dose | Type | Volume/Dose | Type | Volume/Dose |
| Chiasm/optic nerves | Max dose | 10 Gy | Max dose | 17.4 Gy | Max dose | <25 Gy |
| Chiasm/optic nerves | Vol (mL) | <0.2 mL above 8 Gy | Vol (mL) | <0.2 mL above 15.3 Gy | Vol (mL) | <0.2 mL above 23 Gy |
| Ears: Cochlea | Max dose | <9 Gy | Max dose | <17.1 Gy | Max dose | <25 Gy |
| Esophagus | Max dose | <15.4 Gy | Max dose | <25.2 Gy | Max dose | <35 Gy |
| Esophagus | Vol (mL) | <5 mL above 11.9 Gy | Vol (mL) | <5 mL above 17.7 Gy | Vol (mL) | <0.5 mL above 19.5 Gy |
| Eyes: Lens | Max dose | <2 Gy | Max dose | <3 Gy | Max dose | <3 Gy |
| Great vessels | Max dose | <37 Gy | Max dose | <45 Gy | Max dose | <53 Gy |
| Great vessels | Vol (mL) | <10 mL above 31 Gy | Vol (mL) | <10 mL above 39 Gy | Vol (mL) | <10 mL above 47 Gy |
| Heart | Max dose | <22 Gy | Max dose | <30 Gy | Max dose | <38 Gy |
| Heart | Vol (mL) | <15 mL above 16 Gy | Vol (mL) | <15 mL above 24 Gy | Vol (mL) | <15 mL above 32 Gy |
| Liver | Vol to spare | Keep 700 mL <9.1 Gy | Vol to spare | Keep 700 mL <19.2 Gy | Vol to spare | Keep 700 mL <21 Gy |
| Lungs | Mean dose | <6 Gy | Mean dose | <6 Gy | Mean dose | <6 Gy |
| Lungs | Vol to spare | Keep 1,500 mL <7 Gy | Vol to spare | Keep 1,500 mL <11.5 Gy | Vol to spare | Keep 1,500 mL <12.5 Gy |

(continued)

# TABLE A2.2: TISSUE TOLERANCES STEREOTACTIC (CONTINUED)

| Organ | 1 Fraction | | 3 Fractions | | 5 Fractions | |
|---|---|---|---|---|---|---|
| | Type | Volume/Dose | Type | Volume/Dose | Type | Volume/Dose |
| Penile bulb | Max dose | <34 Gy | Max dose | <42 Gy | Max dose | <50 Gy |
| Penile bulb | Vol (mL) | <3 mL above 14 Gy | Vol (mL) | <3 mL above 21.9 Gy | Vol (mL) | <3 mL above 30 Gy |
| Renal cortex | Vol to spare | Keep 200 mL <8.4 Gy | Vol to spare | Keep 200 mL <16 Gy | Vol to spare | Keep 200 mL <17.5 Gy |
| Renal hilum | Vol (%) | <66% <10.6 Gy | Vol (%) | <66% <18.6 Gy | Vol (%) | <66% <23 Gy |
| Sacral plexus | Max dose | <16 Gy | Max dose | <24 Gy | Max dose | <32 Gy |
| Sacral plexus | Vol (mL) | <5 mL above 14.4 Gy | Vol (mL) | <5 mL above 22.5 Gy | Vol (mL) | <5 mL above 30 Gy |
| Skin | Max dose | <26 Gy | Max dose | <33 Gy | Max dose | <39.5 Gy |
| Skin | Vol (mL) | <10 mL above 23 Gy | Vol (mL) | <10 mL above 30 Gy | Vol (mL) | <10 mL above 36.5 Gy |
| Spinal cord | Max dose | <14 Gy | Max dose | <21.9 Gy | Max dose | <30 Gy |
| Spinal cord | Vol (mL) | <0.35 mL above 10 Gy | Vol (mL) | <0.35 mL above 18 Gy | Vol (mL) | <0.35 mL above 23 Gy |
| Spinal cord | Vol (mL) | <1.2 mL above 7 Gy | Vol (mL) | <1.2 mL above 12 Gy | Vol (mL) | <1.2 mL above 14.5 Gy |

# INDEX

Printed in the United States
By Bookmasters